Kiss Your Life Hello with Polysaccharides and Polypeptides

By Dr. Howard Peiper

Kiss Your Life Hello with
Polysaccharides and Polypeptides
Revised

Copyright ©2021
All Rights Reserved
No part of this book may be reproduced in any form
without the written consent of the authors.

Printed in the United States of America
ISBN 9781088005798 ISpark
Library of Congress Control Number: 2021912460
All Rights Reserved

No part of this book may be reproduced in any form
without the written consent of the publisher.

Kiss Your Life Hello with Polysaccharides and Polypeptides is not intended as medical advice, but as suggested complementary therapeutic regimens, to be considered only if deemed adequate by both patients and their chosen health professional. It is written solely for informational and educational purposes.

Safe Goods Publishing
561 Shunpike Rd.
Sheffield, MA 01257
413-229-9042

Table of Contents

	Dedication	5
	Introduction	7
	Foreword	11
One:	Origin and Function	13
Two:	Immune System	19
Three:	Polysaccharides/polypeptides and Anti-Aging	23
Four:	The Brain and Mental Function	33
Five:	Polysaccharides/polypeptides and Diabetes	39
Six:	Polysaccharides/polypeptides for High Cholesterol & Cardiovascular Disease	41
Seven:	Polysaccharides/polypeptides and Cancer	45
Eight:	Polysaccharides/polypeptides and Chronic Fatigue Syndrome	47
Nine:	Polysaccharides/polypeptides and Hepatitis	49
Ten:	Polysaccharides/polypeptides and Arthritis	51
Eleven:	Sports Conditioning and Fatigue	53

Twelve:	Natural Skin Care at the Cellular Level	57
Thirteen:	Research Studies	61
Fourteen:	Frequently Asked Questions	77
Fifteen:	Professional Citations	81
Sixteen:	User Testimonials	87
	Conclusion	107

Dedication

This book is dedicated to a Higher Source who ultimately inspires those scientists, known to them or not, to work hard and be thorough in their research. These gifted men and women have been able to harness the incredible healing power of polysaccharides/polypeptides.

Kiss Your Life Hello with Polysaccharides and Polypeptides.

Introduction

Sit down before a fact as a little child, be prepared to give up every preconceived notion, follow humbly wherever and to whatever abysses nature leads, or you shall learn nothing.
- Thomas Huxley

Nature and science are not always a marriage made in heaven. Until those in the health care profession realize the necessity of a bond between the two, millions of people will continue to suffer and die needlessly. This book is devoted to the benefits of what I believe to be the most powerful of whole food complexes.

It has been said, "The answers to all of man's medical questions and the cures for all ills have been placed on this earth by God. It is just up to us to find them." While this statement might have fallen on deaf ears up to a few years ago, it certainly rings true today. The cultural priorities of technology, progress, and seeking wealth have blinded us from seeing the truth: *To destroy our planet is to destroy the human race.* Coping with water and air pollution, making poor food choices, and entertaining unhealthy lifestyle options may be our sad but inevitable epitaph.

From the common cold to cancer, we have become victims of free radicals, which ultimately wear down our immune system and inhibit its ability to defend and heal our body. These destructive culprits are found everywhere. They originate in food additives, byproducts of plastics, pollution, emotional stress and even sunlight. These unstable oxygen molecules are thought to be largely responsible for the degenerative processes that promote aging and even more importantly, are thought to be the largest contributor of disease. Research has proven that free radicals destroy. We subject ourselves to these killers, sometimes knowingly, and still, we shake our heads and wonder why we develop disease.

What chance do we have against this villain? How do we eliminate these sources of destructive molecules? Improving air quality, purifying water, and improving diet does help. Reducing stress is easier said than done. Even if we attempt to change our lifestyles, we still may fall short of restoring our bodies to good health. Therefore, we must search for other means of combating free radical degeneration. The conventional weapons, called "antioxidants" are not enough.

While physicians have studied and trained hard to make a difference in peoples' lives, modern medicine often fails to achieve total wellness. Allopathic (traditional) medicines have been no match for many life-threatening diseases. Normal cells of the body can mutate into cancer cells and short circuit the immune system. This is possibly mediated by viruses, which may cause the body's defenses to attack themselves. These events have been implicated in diseases such as multiple sclerosis, possibly related to free radical damage. In effect we have become victims, a condition most likely brought about through our own short-sidedness and irresponsibility. Succumbing to our fast-paced lifestyles can result in ever increasing mortality numbers from heart disease, cancer, stroke, and conditions such as high blood pressure, high cholesterol, and diabetes. Is our society creating sufficient awareness of these problems to effectively address them or are we simply too busy trying to survive each day?

Needless to say, the preceding declaration of doom is quite depressing, but all is not lost. The outlook is no longer as hopeless as it once was. In the pages that follow, you will learn of a unique natural food formula unlike any other. It has been widely used for many years in Asia by doctors and other health care providers. It is made from a form of a *whole food complex* that is able to win the battle against free radical destruction—polysaccharides/polypeptides.

Results obtained from its users reveal that polysaccharides/polypeptides can prevent disease, stave off degenerative processes and strengthen the immune system. When ingested polysaccharides/polypeptides can assist the body in healing *at the cellular level*. As a form of a whole-food complex, polysaccharides/polypeptides facilitates the body in taking an active role in healing and impacting the many conditions mediated by the derailment of the immune system. As the pages that follow will show, nature and science have joined together and harnessed polysaccharides/polypeptides. Together they are truly creating miracles.
- *Dr. Howard Peiper*

Kiss Your Life Hello with Polysaccharides and Polypeptides.

Foreword

"Though this is a small book, the information it contains is gigantic. Valuable information offered by Howard Peiper touches the most important aspects of your health. Enjoy your reading experience, through which your life may be enriched. The information provided will allow you to be better prepared to make choices regarding the control of your health.

It is time for a paradigm shift. Our health system is in crisis. The relationship between patients and doctors has been compromised in the name of a third-party liability or insurance. Physicians seem to rely on chemicals (pills) to suppress symptoms, schedule too little time for a comprehensive diagnosis, and are focused on wealth accumulation. These conditions can create confusing scenarios.

Many doctors have little knowledge that minor complaints or symptoms may be caused by an imbalance in the body, a lack of nutrients, or a build-up of toxins. Their solution is to administer symptom-suppressing pills that may calm but rarely cure. Diagnoses, either real or created, are levied for various reasons as being part of the standard medical practice. In doing this, the opportunity of reaching the core of the problem and bringing corrective measures is lost. All this is done under the influence of fear. The patient is fearful of the diagnosis and the doctor is fearful of being wrong, most likely because of potential malpractice claims. Yet, fear is not conducive to healing.

I believe every doctor needs to read this book in order to better understand what alternatives may be available to prescription drugs that continue to silence symptoms without treating the cause. There are many alternatives such as analyzing the patient's acid/alkaline pH, a simple procedure that can offer much information. But yet, this is still far from being incorporated in the evaluation of the patient. Are we looking at the nutritional status of patients? Are we concerned with his or her antioxidant levels? What system of detoxification (ridding the body of toxins) is or could be safely implemented?

This book is a wakeup call; it's time to take control. A doctor's primary responsibility is to the patient, not the insurance or drug company. Reading this book should be an event that is transformational for the patient. Dr. Peiper has given vital and cutting-edge information in a simple format. It is easy to assimilate and incorporate into your choice for protocols when dealing with ill health. It is refreshing to know there is a book that helps the patient relate symptoms to illness and one that offers an alternative to prescriptions that simply suppress those symptoms.

This book is extremely informative. All my patients will be invited to feast on it, and I will make every effort to bring it to as many colleagues as time will permit. It is rewarding to know that there are writers taking the necessary steps to bring sound information to today's society. Howard, I am grateful for your research. May the good Lord give you His many blessings.

-*Esteban Genao, MD, FAAP*

Chapter One

Origin and Function

Rice is the culinary culture as well the basis for economical solvency in many societies. For example, the Burmese cultural history embraces ancient folklore where the Kachins people of northern Myanmar were sent forth from the center of the Earth with seeds of rice. These people were directed to a wondrous country where everything was perfect and where rice grew well. Today rice remains as their leading crop and a most revered food. In Bali, it is believed that the Lord Vishnu caused the Earth to give birth to rice, and the God Indra taught the people how to raise it. In both myths rice is considered a gift of the gods. Even in modern times the people of both countries treat rice with its according reverence and its cultivation is tied to elaborate rituals.

By contrast, a Thai myth tells of rice being a gift of animals rather than of gods. This was a time when Thailand had been engulfed by severe weather and wracked with floods. After the land finally drained, people came down from the hills where they had taken refuge only to discover that all the plants had been destroyed and there was little to eat. They survived through hunting although animals were scarce. According to the writings, one day the people saw a dog coming across a field and hanging on the dog's tail were bunches of long, yellow seeds. They planted these seeds. Rice grew, and hunger disappeared. Throughout Thailand today, tradition holds that "the precious things are not pearls and jade but are the five grains," of which rice is the first. While most modern Thai's may intellectually dismiss its supernatural role, they cannot deny the enormous cultural importance of rice in their country, and also in most of the other rice-producing and rice-consuming countries of the world.

Science Meets Myth

Scientists have utilized ancient Thai folk medicine, techniques, and theory, combined with modern and sophisticated technology to produce polysaccharide/polypeptides. Alphaglycanology is a proprietary and innovative process employing biotechnology and nanotechnology. The purpose of the Alphaglycanology technique is to mechanically hydrolyze polysaccharides[1] and polypeptides[2] in cereal grains, from specially selected fractions of rice grains, harvested at the proper age. The grain is grown in an area where the soils are alkaline in nature and continuously enriched with natural organic matter containing abundant spirulina[3] found in the water. The rice is organically grown, free of pesticides and insecticides and is not modified in any way.

By bonding the polysaccharides/polypeptides together under controlled humidity, temperature and pressure, a naturally hydrolyzed alpha-glycan is formed. Thus, producing an incredibly beneficial functional food. When consumed, it is recognized by the cells of the body as a biological fuel for utilization by the mitochondria for the production of cellular energy or ATP (adenosine triphosphate). A recent study demonstrated a significant increase of ATP in mitochondria metabolism of 54 percent.

The special characteristics of polysaccharides/polypeptides, produced with the Alphaglycanology process, allows for 100 percent bioavailability.[4] When consumed, these unique functional genomic nutrients are readily assimilated facilitating an improvement of the intracellular environment. This is essential for DNA repair and the resulting enhanced gene expression. Correspondingly, the environment manifested in the body is vitally essential for optimal health. The alphaglycanology process em-

---

[1] any of the more complex carbohydrates
[2] molecular chain of amino acids
[3] a superior source of essential nutrients and antioxidants
[4] total absorption on a cellular level

ployed by scientists to produce the polysaccharides/polypeptides has shown its ability to effectively preserve the functional value of the phytonutrients.

Scientists have found that when certain species of rice grains are grown under optimal conditions, and are harvested at the proper age, they contain top quality functional and essential nutrients such as specific polysaccharides, polypeptides, the amino acids, vitamins, minerals, and antioxidants (gamma oryzanol, tocopherol tocotrienols). Rice grains meeting these criteria are perfectly suited to enhance the cellular energy (ATP) production of the mitochondria for DNA repair and cellular regeneration. They can combat free radicals and enhance the detoxification process establishing an anabolic (building) phase so that the body's natural healing power may function optimally. The unique combination of these antioxidants, organic mineral amino acid compounds, and polysaccharides, has the ability to stimulate the body to naturally regulate a state of *homeostasis* (when the body is in balance). This results in balanced levels of blood sugar, cholesterol, triglycerides, blood pressure, body temperature, electrolytes, and pH.

There are several different sources of polysaccharides/polypeptides: aloe vera, medicinal mushrooms (reishi, maitake, shiitake), and nutritional primary yeast. Below is the difference between a beta-glucan polysaccharide/polypeptide and an alpha-glycan processed polysaccharide/polypeptide.

Alpha-Glucan (Glycan) vs. Beta-Glucan

Alpha-Glucan (Glycan) linkages can be easily broken down by alpha-amylase. Therefore, single units of glucose and amino acid can be utilized by cells and white blood cells. Glucose will be used to produce energy (ATP). With energy and the correct type of amino acid, white blood cells will have all the necessary raw materials to produce a certain type of antibody whenever foreign materials enter our body. While there is no foreign material, cells can use energy and the correct type of amino acid for improving normal repairing process.

Beta-glucan is highly soluble, but the beta linkage is difficult to break down due to the limited amount of glucoamylase. Beta-glucan acts as a foreign material. It touches the receptor and stimulates white blood cells to generate a certain type of antibody. This is a process that requires energy and the correct type of amino acid from our body. If the body does not have enough energy and/or the correct type of amino acid, the production process for a certain type of antibody is not effective. If the production of a certain type of antibody is too effective and generates excessive antibody while there is an absence of foreign material, some undesirable symptoms might occur.

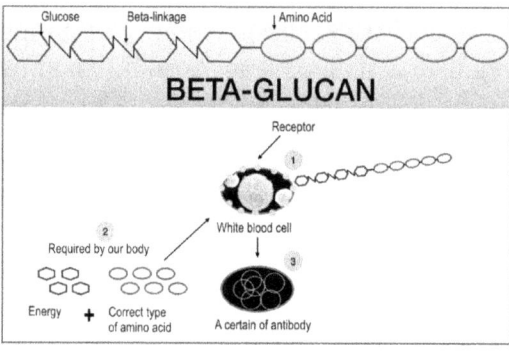

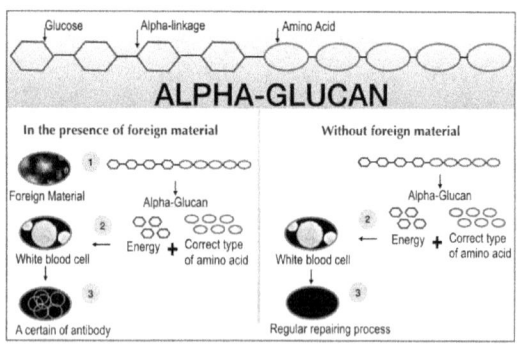

pH Balance

The scale used to measure the body's acidity and alkalinity is called pH, normally measured in a range from one to fourteen. A neutral solution, neither acidic nor alkaline, has a pH of seven; acid is less than seven, alkaline is more than seven. The blood must be kept within the very narrow range of pH 7.4 to maintain homeostasis (balance).

Unfortunately, the average North American diet is very high in acid foods, such as sugar, refined carbohydrates and starch. These are not conducive to maintaining proper pH balance in the body and raise acid levels. To prevent disease from getting a foothold in this acid environment it is imperative that homeostasis be restored, which can be accomplished by adding trace minerals to the diet. This acidic condition is caused by metabolic waste. When trace minerals are in sufficient quantity they bind with the waste and flush it out through the urine thus returning the body to a more balanced state.

Excessive acid waste literally attacks the joints, tissues, muscles, organs, and glands, causing minor to major dysfunction. If it affects the joints, arthritis may develop; effects on the muscles may result in myofibrosis (aching muscles); attacks on the organs and glands, can cause a myriad of illnesses. The more acidic the body is, the more compromised the immune system becomes. A constant diet of foods excessively high in protein and sugar results in a more acidic body and weakens the immune system allowing conditions like chronic fatigue syndrome, cancer, MS, and arthritis to gain a foothold.

pH-balancing the body slightly more on the alkaline side than on the acid should be a daily goal. Because polysaccharides/polypeptides are made from a whole food that is grown in an alkalized, mineral-enriched environment, it has the ability to facilitate a slightly alkaline pH balance. When the pH is balanced in the body, it is able to totally absorb all nutrients from foods and supplements. Polysaccharides/polypeptides efficiently creates and maintains a pH-balanced body.

Detoxification
An important function of polysaccharides/polypeptides is its ability to detoxify[5] the body. Avoiding contact with toxins on a daily basis is virtually impossible, and a buildup of these toxins within the body results in many forms of illness. Cleanliness, externally and internally, is essential to good health. Polysaccharides/polypeptides assist this process because it works on the entire body to remove toxins from the system. When these toxins are eliminated polysaccharides/polypeptides help support and strengthen the glandular system helping the body heal itself.

The colon and the bowel become the depository for all waste material after food nutrients are extracted into the bloodstream. Decaying food ferments and forms gases as well as second and even third generation toxins. Thus, the colon becomes a breeding ground for putrefactive bacteria, viruses, parasites, yeast and more. Because of polysaccharides/polypeptides fiber-like structure the peristalsis movement of the colon is strengthened, and bowel movements are healthier and more regular, better facilitating the elimination process. Healthy intestines are the body's second immune system. Therefore, it is essential to keep them free of putrefied waste.

---

[5] to remove a poison or toxin

Chapter Two

The Immune System

> *No illness which can be treated by diet should be treated by any other means.*
> –Moses Maimonides, the great physician of 12th century

The immune system's basic function is to protect us against infection, illness and disease of all kinds. It fights off thousands of predatory environmental and infectious microorganisms, which can invade and damage virtually every part of the body. The immune system' function is to expel pathogens (virus' bacteria, etc.), toxic chemicals, and tumorous cells that are generated through mutation. It also aids the body in tissue repair and healing and strives to maintain homeostasis (balance) in the body.

The immune system involves a finely tuned, highly integrated series of events that destroy a would-be invader. Once the immune system identifies an unwanted guest, it brings an awesome array of chemical and cellular weapons to banish the perpetrators. This non-specific, intricate, and elaborate immune response can readily discriminate between the "self" and "non-self", that is, cells that are a normal part of the body versus alien organisms. The innate intelligence of the immune system insures that the body does not turn on itself and lose the ability to distinguish between the "good and bad" cells.

Autoimmunity

When the immune system loses the ability to distinguish between self and non-self it may develop an autoimmunity (the body manufacturing antibodies and T-cells directed against its own cells, cell components or even specific organs). Autoimmune responses include allergies, asthma, rheumatoid arthritis, dermatitis, diabetes, systemic lupus erythematosis, multiple sclerosis, fibromyalgia and also may be the underlying factor in numerous chronic conditions. When the body is under constant exposure to various pathogens the immune system will become over stimulated resulting in autoimmunity.

Weakened Immunity
When the immune system is working properly we remain healthy. However, the immune system can and does become compromised. This may be a result of the following: incessant environmental assault such as from exposure to pseudo-estrogens; pesticides and pollutants in air, food and water; certain medications; persistent metabolic damage, (for example, high free-radical stress); poor nutrition, chronic infection or advancing age; and strenuous physical activity and emotional stress. As you can see, numerous diverse factors may compromise the immune system and disturb its exquisitely balanced components.

It is no secret that our body is put under physical and emotional stress warding off the above-mentioned multi-faceted assaults. When our bodies become overwhelmed, the regulatory features of the immune system weaken and become less effective resulting in fatigue, loss of stamina and energy, frequent colds and infections, loss of appetite and weight loss, fever and night sweats, skin rashes and cold sores, diarrhea, increased severity of allergy symptoms, swollen lymph nodes, and other symptoms of immune deficiencies.

In time, these conditions can exacerbate the initial symptoms into more serious immuno-compromised conditions (such as chronic fatigue, cancer, HIV, etc.). It is widely believed that cancer may be caused by a decline in the immune system function attributed to aging, lifestyle and other factors. The AIDS virus is known to destroy our immune cells and trigger a multitude of bodily system breakdowns.

Over time, normal cell-mediated immunity may become inadequate or malfunction. This may allow multiple genetic mutations in the same location (malignant transformations) resulting in abnormal growth. The degenerative process is generally quite slow and elusive. It may take many years and many bouts of illness to truly manifest itself where a diagnosis is levied.

Polysaccharides/polypeptides have strong immune-stimulating properties. Health care practitioners have consistently observed the therapeutic benefits produced by polysaccharides and polypeptides for a wide range of health problems. It has been shown to promote vast improvement in cases of many common but serious health problems, ranging from cancer, chronic fatigue syndrome, high blood pressure, rheumatoid arthritis, Parkinson's, Alzheimer's, diabetes, hepatitis, high cholesterol, tumors, Tourette's, irritable bowel syndrome.[6]

To maintain good health, minimize the frequency and severity of all illnesses, and recover quickly, it is imperative that the immune system function efficiently and optimally. The more hazards we expose the body to, the greater the call for the immune system to maintain our health. Natural immune support is very important, making dietary additions such as polysaccharides/polypeptides a primary consideration.

---

[6] Ishak, Dr. Mohammed, "Possible Solutions to the Global Health Problems," *Nature's Journal*, April 2002.

Kiss Your Life Hello with Polysaccharides and Polypeptides.

Chapter Three

Polysaccharides/polypeptides and Anti-Aging

Aging—it's happening to everybody. Time is accelerating the aging process faster than we'd like. Even though the hourglass tells us we're older the passage of time isn't really what ages us. The aging culprit is the process that creates a reduction of healthy cells in our body.

Cells don't age; they're sloughed off as their efficiency diminishes and are replaced by new ones. With proper nutrition cell restoration continues in excess of what is generally considered a normal life expectancy. Industrialized civilization breeds environmental pollutants, diets full of chemicals and additives, vitamin and mineral deficiencies, and the overuse of prescription drugs. This menu of assaults gives rise to an early retirement in the cemetery. Today, industrialized countries boast statistics that claim 80 percent of the population over the age of sixty-five years old is chronically ill, usually with arthritis, diabetes or high blood pressure.[7]

The key to long life is emotional and physical balance (homeostasis). Our general loss of vitality and disease originate from poor diet, life-style choices, or from long-term environmental assaults. Yet, there is hope. Youthfulness is restored from the inside, by strengthening our lean body mass, metabolism, and immune response with good nutrition, regular exercise, fresh air, and a positive mental attitude.

---

[7] Page, Linda, ND, PhD, *Healthy Healing 11th Edition*, Traditional Wisdom, 2000.

Fountain of Youth

Through my research I have determined that polysaccharides/polypeptides can play a big role in our search for the "fountain of youth." The antioxidant properties of polysaccharides/polypeptides prevent body components from destruction by free radicals—a key to anti-aging.

The three important contributors to aging are: cell and tissue damage caused by free radicals;[8] reduced immune response, and enzyme depletion in the body due to diets composed of enzyme deficient foods (cooked or processed.)

Free radicals, (highly active compounds produced when molecules react with oxygen,) play a key role in the deterioration of the body. Under assault from chemicalized foods and environmental pollutants, our bodies generate excesses of these cell damagers. After years of free-radical assaults cells become irreplaceably lost from major organs such as the lungs, liver, kidneys, the brain, and particularly our nervous system. This loss is seen as a primary cause of aging.

Alzheimer's, Parkinson's, and Multiple Sclerosis are thought to be associated with the aging process due to three potent neurotoxins, Beta-Amyloid, Glutamate, and Peroxides, that can lead to nerve cell damage and destruction. These molecules disrupt and destroy normal nerve cell function.

Studies reveal those polysaccharides/polypeptides have been shown to preserve nerve cell function by supplying food and nutrients at the cellular level. The concept is simple. Provide the cell with food easily recognized and utilized by the cell's DNA (the "molecule of life") to generate energy. This will provide the vehicle for repairing cell damage.

This is incredible news for people with Alzheimer's and Creutzfeldt-Jakob diseases. Both illnesses manifest when a neurotoxin, called Beta Amyloid, deposits itself in the brain and disrupts

---

[8] unstable fragments of molecules produced from oxygen and fats in cells

communication between nerve cells. Scientists have tried to treat the diseases by attacking the protein deposits but to date this approach has not been successful.

A new study shows that by helping nerve cells produce normal proteins these connections can actually be rejuvenated.[9] In this study, nerve cells exposed to three of the most potent neurotoxins were ultimately protected from damage after adding polysaccharides/polypeptides to the medium. A degree of cellular regeneration of the nerve dendrites and axons was also seen. These extraordinary results have consistently been observed in subsequent research.

Superoxide dismutase (SOD) is an extremely potent antioxidant enzyme that fights cellular damage from single oxygen molecules (also known as free radicals). As an enzyme, SOD has particular value in helping to protect against cell destruction. Research suggests that SOD may be the most important enzyme in the body for the control of free radicals, keeping our cell membranes young, supple, and healthy (anti-aging). Although SOD has been sold as a supplement, research shows that oral SOD is destroyed by the digestive system before it can fight free radicals and repair damaged joints. This suggests that the most viable means of building healthy levels of SOD in the body would be to consume natural food substances that bind protein to SOD and therefore deliver it via the digestive system to the body, without being destroyed in the gut. Polysaccharides/polypeptides facilitates that process and increases the level of SOD in the body.

There are numerous antioxidants[10] made by the body as well as antioxidants found through supplementation or in

---

[9] Sawatsri, Sayan, MD, Yankunthong, Wanphen, M.Sc, *Polysaccharides/polypeptices may Prevent Neuron Vulnerablility in Human Neuroblastoma Cells,* PMK Research Institute, Bangkok, Thailand, March, 2001.

[10] a substance that inhibits oxidation or reactions promoted by oxygen or peroxides

our diets. Nutrients like vitamins E and C, beta-carotene and the trace mineral selenium root out any free radicals that make it past the antioxidant enzymes. It is necessary to support the body's own production of antioxidant enzymes (SOD) because they remove free radicals three to ten times faster than the nutrient antioxidants. The body will benefit far more if it can produce its own antioxidant enzymes, and that is what polysaccharides and polypeptides facilitates.

Polysaccharides/polypeptides is a premier agent for reversing the causes of aging by utilizing the following:
1. Increasing the level of SOD (superoxide dismutase), the master antioxidant;
2. Enhancing nucleotide production for DNA repair;
3. Enhancing cellular environment for improved genetic expression;
4. Increasing pro-enzyme and probiotic (friendly intestinal bacteria) activities.

"Since I started taking polysaccharides/polypeptides my sexual performance has been enhanced. I am sixty-one years old, in a relationship with a 44-year-old female and was dismayed when I found my sexual energy diminishing. I had thought of taking *Viagra*. However, my Naturopathic Doctor suggested trying polysaccharides/polypeptides. It worked and I am so grateful that I listened to him."
-*Julio Cabral, Mexico City, Mexico*

Slowing the Aging Process
Aging is an inherent part of life's great cycle. Yet, as natural as it is to age, so is it natural to wonder how we can avoid the seemingly inevitable decline that comes with aging. Must the wisdom and grace won by living be spoiled by a loss of comfort, mobility,

and power to achieve? Must health and strength disappear just when we are getting the hang of life? We hear reports of "exceptional" people - farmers in northern climates, saints in eastern mountains – who live with vitality and vigor far past the century mark. We instinctively sense that they are living the most natural lives of all. And so, we wonder: Is it possible that aging's negative effects are not inevitable at all, and that deep within our cells we have a capacity for infinite renewal?

To meet an ever-growing demand for longer and healthier life, researchers all over the world are striving to unlock the secrets of longevity. As they begin to uncover the causes of age-related decline, they are discovering new ways to prevent premature aging. Their findings have yielded many approaches: dietary changes, exercise, special supplements, and others. Yet the essential questions remain. What makes our bodies and minds wear out? And perhaps more pressing, how can we reverse the negative effects of aging or even prevent them altogether?

What Happens When We Age?

When we are vibrantly healthy, our body's cells are functioning at their peak. They use nutrients and eliminate wastes efficiently, and they contribute fully to the health of the entire organism. We can say that a healthy cell is one that is doing a good job of following the "blueprint" for how it is supposed to work.

Indeed, within every cell lies its blueprint for optimal health. Of course, unlike an architect's blueprint, a cell's blueprint is not a physical drawing. Instead, it is a pattern of energy frequencies. This pattern provides the cell with an ideal picture of how it should function and how to repair itself when needed. The information in our cell's blueprints allows us to heal from anything – whether it is the flu, a paper cut, pneumonia, cancer, sunburn, or a broken heart.

As we age, cells tend to forget and stray from their blueprints. Over a lifetime, as we experience times of less-than-ideal nutrition, emotional ups and downs, environmental toxins, and the general stress of living, these experiences leave their marks on our cells. These cellular deposits are both physical and energetic. They obstruct the cells' vision of their blueprints. When the cells cannot read their blueprints clearly, they naturally begin to stray from them.

When cells stray from their blueprints, the cells functioning, and structure move away from the ideal. Dysfunction, illness, and premature aging begin to set in. The body's natural flexibility and adaptability – that is, its ability to respond to and recover from stresses – diminishes. Therefore, anything that (1) helps cells regain their awareness of their natural blueprints, and (2) restores the body's flexibility and adaptability will foster health and longevity.

Introducing PSP

PSP (polysaccharides/polypeptides)is a nutritional food that has the extraordinary ability to reawaken our cells to their blueprints. It keeps the cells attention focused on their blueprints and thus helps reestablish the cells' adaptability. This effectively reverses the negative effects of aging and lets us tap into our inner reservoir of radiant vitality.

Leading Cells Toward Their Blueprints

Unhealthy cells are like a person in a dark forest who cannot see the path that could lead back into the sunshine. Like a compass pointing north. PSP turns the cells attention toward their blueprints so that they can see their way out of their predicament. When the cells become aware of their blueprints, they are reminded of their highest potential for health. They can see what they are aiming for. Given this chance, the cells naturally and spontaneously work to maintain the highest degree of health possible.

Energetic Cells: The Opposite of Aging

To understand how PSP helps keep the cells attention on their blueprint, let us look a little deeper – at the atoms that make up our cells, and hence our bodies. Modern physics teaches us that atomic particles can switch constantly between states of matter and energy. When the atomic particles that compromise the body are in an energy state, the body naturally takes on more properties of energy. The body becomes more fluid, adaptable, and open to the free flow of life energy. This life energy nourishes and invigorates the cells, allowing the body to evolve and repair itself.

Yet, as our bodies age or become diseased, their atoms spend more and more time in the matter state. The body's vibrations become denser. The movement of its atoms slows down, and they become more static. When the cells atoms spend most of the time in the more rigid matter state, the cells lose their adaptability, and they gradually deteriorate and age. Hardness and rigidity set in, which prevents the free flow of energy. Perhaps most important, cells become unable to "read" and follow their blueprints for optimal health.

Consequently, one secret to maintaining youth is to keep our atoms in an energy state as much, and as long, as possible. PSP can help us do this through its extraordinary ability to help produce *energy* in the body. Because of the fluidity and flexibility that characterize the energy state, we can say that when most of a cell's atoms are in an energy state, the cell achieves a state of energetic abundance. Thus, the more energy a cell has, the more easily it can adapt and evolve toward greater health. It helps puts cells in the direction of optimal health.

The Benefits are Many

Recall that the cells blueprints are patterns of energy frequencies. Because energetic cells have more properties, they resonate more easily with the energetic frequencies of the blueprints. This resonance allows them to read and follow the blueprints more easily and accurately. For the same reason, energetic cells can also gather more life energy directly from the environment, as they need it.

Because in an energy state, space becomes more flexible, energetic cells can also communicate with other energetic cells in the body directly. Thus, they easily exchange information about nutrients, energy management, and needed repairs. Areas comprised of energetic cells are also relaxed, yet highly dynamic. Like Olympic athletes, masters at remaining relaxed while their muscles are working at peak capacity, energetic areas are restful and consume little energy, yet are ready at any moment to spring into action at an optimal level. As more and more of the body achieves energy, one feels more vital, strong, fluid, and alive.

Holistic Microscopy: Live and Dry Blood demonstration by Fred Shadian

Client: Female
Age: 57
Lifestyle: Vegetarian
Test Time: 21 Days (3 weeks)
Amount of VidaCell: 2 to 3 packets per day

*Below are pictures of the client's best Live and Dry blood samples taken on Saturday January 5, 2008.

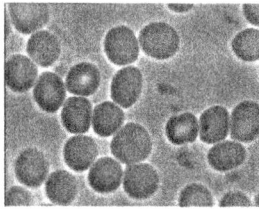 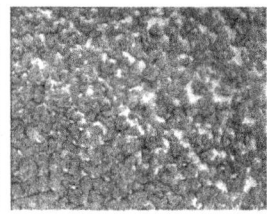

---
*Below are pictures of the client's best Live and Dry blood samples taken 21 days later on Saturday January 28, 2008.

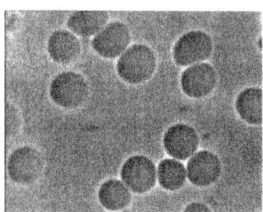 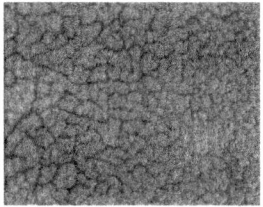

Kiss Your Life Hello with Polysaccharides and Polypeptides.

Chapter Four

The Brain and Mental Function

The brain is a delicate and complex structure. As the control center of all physical and intellectual activity in the body it utilizes as many as 100 billion different cells, with millions and millions of neurons forming a seemingly innumerable number of connections. It is responsible for all of our internal functions and our interactions with our external surroundings. In order to maintain this relationship, the brain must be functioning properly. For us to enjoy life to the fullest, we need to be in control. Optimal functioning is desired for optimal interaction. Around the age of thirty, neurons (brain cells) begin to die (or go dormant). After this age, they die at a faster rate than they are replaced, thus beginning the degenerative process that becomes more and more obvious as we get older.

Neurons are large cells, which require large amounts of energy and proper nutrition to function normally. The brain receives 15-20 percent of the body's total blood supply and uses 15-20 percent of the body's total inhaled oxygen, which along with glucose, is used by the brain to produce and use 15-20 percent of the body's total ATP (adenosine triphosphate) energy. Unlike most other cells, which can burn fat or glucose for their energy needs, neurons can only burn glucose. Under normal conditions our brain cells typically consume 50 percent of the total blood glucose. Therefore, neurons and cells in the brain are dependent upon a continuous and uninterrupted rich blood supply to maintain normal energy metabolism and avoid cellular injury or death.

Under normal conditions, with adequate oxygen supply, these neurons convert glucose into (ATP) for three reasons:

1. Cell maintenance: Since neurons don't reproduce and must last a lifetime, they are continually expending energy to repair or replace various cell parts—cell membrane segments, microtubules, mitochondria, etc.
2. Neurotransmitter operation: Neurons use ATP to produce, transport, package, secrete, and re-uptake neurotransmitters such as acetylcholine and serotonin, which provide vital cell-to-cell communication.
3. Electrical energy: Huge amounts of ATP are necessary to facilitate the frequent discharges of electrical energy from the neuron through the cell body to the transmitting end—the axon. For this electrical process to occur there must be a rapid and continuous exchange of sodium and potassium ions back and forth across the neuronal membranes.

Over a lifetime, there can be slow and subtle memory loss resulting from brain-energy losses due to cerebral arteriosclerosis, ministrokes, neurotoxins (glutamate, beta-amyloid, and peroxides), or brief interruptions of brain oxygen supply (often caused by blood vessel spasm). In addition to memory impairment, this brain energy crisis may also cause occasional confusion or lapses in concentration and learning difficulties.

For reasons we are only beginning to understand the neuron-replacement process is far more evident in some people than in others. One octogenarian will be fully self-sufficient, remembering not only what they need to do for that day, but also the details of some event that happened over forty years ago. However, others may not remember their own telephone number or the names of their children or grandchildren.

At a more advanced stage the brain energy crisis may show itself as senility or senile dementia, and eventually may terminate in coma or death. The severity of dementia is directly correlated to the loss of functional brain tissue independent of the primary neuropathology. If someone's brain is not working correctly it is largely because of brain disease (such as Alzheimer's, Parkinson's, brain tumor, infection, vascular disturbances), injury (such as from brain trauma, stroke, stress, neurotoxins, alcohol or drugs), or deficiencies of EFA's (essential fatty acids) or B complex vitamins.

Symptoms of Cognitive Deterioration
Cognitive deterioration can involve the loss or decline of any of the cognitive functions including:
- Memory
- Orientation
- Information fixation
- Attention
- Perception
- Judgment

Major contributing factors to cognitive degeneration may include the following:
- Chronic circulatory problems in the brain: This includes a variety of medical conditions that decrease the delivery of blood flow to the brain reducing glucose, oxygen, and nutrients to the brain cells;
- Various cerebral disorders: These include Alzheimer's or Parkinson's diseases;
- Cerebral hemorrhage;
- Transient ischaemic attacks (TIA): an interrupted blood flow to the brain;
- Various brain-toxic substances: We cite examples such as alcohol, opiates, (morphine, heroin), cocaine, amphetamines, hallucinogens, (STP, LSD, marijuana, etc.) and neurotoxins (glutamate, beta-amyloid and peroxides);
- Various prescribed medications: These may be very toxic to the brain and may cause memory loss, confusion or depression, and may have an adverse effect on brain function. Various prescription medications can include:

pain killers, antidepressants, tranquilizers, sleeping pills, antihistamines, corticosteroids, heart and blood pressure medication.

Individuals with vascular disease or dementia attributed to Alzheimer's often have a disturbance in antioxidant balance that may predispose one to increased oxidative stress. This would then be a potential therapeutic area for antioxidant supplementation.

Enhanced memory function
Polysaccharides/polypeptides are recommended for cerebral circulatory disorders such as memory problems, acute stroke, aphasia (loss of the power of expression), apraxia (inability to coordinate movements), motor disorders, dizziness and other cerebro-vestibular (inner-ear) problems, and headache. Polysaccharides and polypeptides can often be beneficial for acute or chronic ophthalmologic diseases of various origins and may improve vision. Polysaccharides/polypeptides also have a very powerful stimulating effect on memory because of its effect on the brain's metabolism.

Polysaccharides/polypeptides increase the metabolism in the brain several ways:
- It increases the rate at which brain cells produce ATP (which is the cell molecule that creates energy);
- It speeds up the use of glucose in the brain;
- It speeds up the use of oxygen in the brain.

The result is that the cells of the brain can better retain information causing the individual to remember more. Polysaccharides/polypeptides have been reported as showing promising benefits for the following conditions:
- stroke
- vertigo
- Meniere's Syndrome
- depression
- tinnitus
- migraine headaches

- sleep disorders
- mood changes
- Tourette's Syndrome
- ADD/ADHD
- macular degeneration
- convulsions
- Multiple Sclerosis
- Cerebral Palsy

Polysaccharides/polypeptides Increases Neurotransmitters
Polysaccharides/polypeptides stimulate cognitive enhancement primarily through its influence on important neurotransmitters. These neurotransmitters relay information between neurons and rely on specialized brain chemicals to function properly. While memory is an extremely complex phenomenon, neuronal transmission is even more complex. There are more than one hundred different neurotransmitters that have been identified.

Depressed levels of certain neurotransmitters are associated with psychiatric disorders. Depression has been linked with depressed levels of serotonin and Parkinson's has been linked with depressed levels of dopamine. An overabundance of dopamine is associated with Tourette's syndrome (an involuntary movement and vocal disorder, often socially disabling).

Neurotransmitters are responsible for the transmission of information between neurons, indicating that they are necessary for *all* cognitive functions. Polysaccharides/polypeptides support neuronal transmission by:

- increasing levels of noradrenaline (thinking, learning planning);
- balancing levels of dopamine (libido, information processing);
- increasing levels of acetylcholine (memory);
- increasing levels of serotonin (mood, sleep, balances appetite, lowers substance cravings).

Please take note that depression is a symptom of insufficient serotonin levels, which is often caused by prolonged exposure to stressors. Scientists have found that a positive therapeutic effect of polysaccharides/polypeptides was shown in patients who exhibited pronounced depressive states of varied origins. In a recent study, a substantial decrease or complete disappearance of the clinical manifestation of depression was noted in 65 percent of the patients. Serotonin has the ability to help the body adapt to stress. Polysaccharides/polypeptides can raise serotonin levels thereby helping the body resist chronic stress and mood disorders related to low levels of serotonin.

"I cannot say enough good things about this miraculous food. For nine years I had suffered from Multiple Sclerosis experiencing vision problems, muscle weakness, fatigue, dizziness, and burning sensations in my feet. After taking polysaccharides/polypeptides three times a day for several months, all of my symptoms disappeared. I am able to walk without a limp and climb stairs without the aid of a railing. I feel like I have truly found a miracle in my life."

-*Paula Barnes, Washington State*

Chapter Five

Polysaccharides/polypeptides and Diabetes

America is in the midst of a growing epidemic that now affects more than 18 million people. The medical pharmaceutical industry calls this metabolic disorder "diabetes" which occurs when the body is unable to properly utilize insulin, which is designed to help regulate glucose or blood sugar levels in the body. If blood sugar concentrations rise, a number of critical body functions are affected such as metabolism, fluid retention, blood-sugar regulation, and liver function. When the body produces too much insulin and loses its ability to respond appropriately a condition develops known as insulin resistance syndrome. It is estimated that nearly 80 million Americans have this problem, and most of them don't even know it.

Polysaccharides/polypeptides work at the cellular and molecular level providing each and every cell with the energy it needs to metabolize glucose, rid the body of toxins and waste products, and begin cellular regeneration. The molecular structure of polysaccharides/polypeptides allows for improved absorption and assimilation of glucose through direct absorption into the cell. The properties in polysaccharides/polypeptides help keep the glucose-energy metabolism system finely tuned. This dramatically decreases the workload of the liver by enhancing direct cellular absorption of glucose, reducing the amount of insulin release and therefore decreasing the risk of other metabolic disorders.

Polysaccharides/polypeptides will improve health conditions linked with diabetes. For example, one may experience:
- better balance of blood glucose;
- reduced fatigue and more energy;

- enhanced natural production of antioxidants to reduce free radical damage;
- less damage to glucose/energy metabolism;
- better healing of diabetic gangrene, greatly reducing the risk of amputation.

"L.H., age sixty-nine, is amazed that he can walk from his bed to the bathroom without excruciating pain. Since being diagnosed Type II Diabetic in 1993, L.H. has suffered burning and painful tingling sensations in his toes and feet. He experienced such pain that he couldn't bear to walk even the short distance to the bathroom without something on his feet. Like most of us L.H. was very skeptical of the restorative properties of polysaccharides/polypeptides. The pain in his feet and the daily annoyance of taking up to five pills to control his blood sugar prompted him to give polysaccharides/polypeptides a try. Is he ever glad he did! After just three weeks of taking only one scoop a day in the morning, L.H. has cut out his medication by 75 percent. Not only has his blood sugar stabilized, now he has enough energy to go to the gym. Perhaps best of all, he walks with much less pain than before taking polysaccharides/polypeptides."
-*Tien Huynh, New Orleans, LA*

"I've had serious health problems during the last ten years, including Type II Diabetes and colds that would develop into walking pneumonia. Allergic reactions to antibiotics made it all the more difficult to control the illnesses. At the beginning of 2003 I was told about a new whole food supplement called polysaccharides/polypeptides which I began taking in a cup of green tea.

I have had circulation problems for years and although the condition has improved, my feet were still numb and cold to the touch. My remedy for this was to apply *Vicks Vapor Rub* on my feet and wear socks to keep them warm. It helped but didn't solve the problem. I was quite surprised at what happened on the second day of using polysaccharides/polypeptides when I realized that I had forgotten to use the *Vicks*. My feet started itching and I couldn't stop moving my toes and rubbing my feet together. It was evident that the circulation was returning to my feet, and they were healing! I was excited because I feared my circulation problems might lead to serious complications, common in diabetics.

After reporting my newfound 'cure' to my doctor in Las Colinas, he said that he would monitor my progress and reduce my medication if needed. I checked my blood pressure and blood glucose twice a day and noticed that my blood pressure had dropped the first day I took polysaccharides/polypeptides . The average for the last two weeks was 122/68 (had previously tested at 131/88) and my blood glucose average for two weeks was 111 and had been 128. When I was first diagnosed with Type II Diabetes there were times when my eyesight would blur, and I was unable to focus. After taking polysaccharides/polypeptides, I find I rarely use glasses now for reading or writing.

I had been on polysaccharides/polypeptides for six weeks and noticed many changes. I was now free of rashes from allergies. The brown spots on my arms and hands were fading, my eyebrows were growing thicker and there was a marked improvement in my digestion. My metabolism must have increased because I lost inches. My break-through came during the second week after I began taking polysaccharides/polypeptides. I often use a full-body vibrator with heat and never felt the vibration in my ankles and feet until now. I now also find that my energy is unbelievably strong."

-*Donna Marshall, Grand Prairie, TX*

Kiss Your Life Hello with Polysaccharides and Polypeptides.

Chapter Six

Polysaccharides/polypeptides for High Cholesterol and Cardiovascular Disease

According to recent data, over 36 million Americans have a total serum cholesterol count of over 240, which puts them at risk for coronary heart and cardiovascular disease (heart attacks, angina,). Coronary heart disease refers to heart damage that occurs when the coronary arteries become blocked or narrowed due to a buildup of plaque or oxidized cholesterol. For men and women whose cholesterol count falls in the range of 200-240, as it does for over 54 million people, the risk of heart disease is double that of those individuals whose cholesterol levels indicate below 200.

Genetic predisposition and the measured ratio of LDL cholesterol to HDL may determine who will develop coronary disease. However, high total cholesterol is considered a major indicator of potential cardiovascular disease, and can also contribute to gallstones, impotence, mental impairment and hypertension. Even more serious is the risk for cholesterol buildup to break off and lodge in the heart or the brain causing heart attack or stroke.

A study performed at Cho-ray hospital in Vietnam was conducted with three hundred doctors and nurses who have experienced some type of heart condition.[11] They participated in a ninety-day test in which they supplemented their diets with polysaccharides/polypeptides on a daily basis. The results were astonishing. Within the test period, 100 percent of the subjects showed significant improvement in their heart conditions. They are now

---

[11] Cho-Ray Hospital in Hanoi, Vietnam, Study conducted by J.Toan, MD, March 2003.

administering polysaccharides/polypeptides to all of their intensive care unit patients. This study revealed that polysaccharides/polypeptides had a powerful effect on cellular function, which produced:
- lower LDL cholesterol;
- increased HDL cholesterol;
- decreased hypertension;
- reduced apolipoprotein-B (complexes of fat and protein found in blood plasma);
- better ratio of LDL to HDL;
- lower risk of heart attack.

Terry Johnson, from Michigan, had a high cholesterol level and was unable to take the vast number of conventional medications prescribed for her. She was introduced to polysaccharides/polypeptides and gave this report. "After taking polysaccharides/polypeptides for six weeks, my cholesterol level dropped from 318 to 225. My doctor was pleased and advised that I should continue taking it."

Chapter Seven

Polysaccharides/polypeptides and Cancer

Cancer high-risk groups are generally linked to genetics and age, although stress is currently being considered a contributor because it weakens the immune system and makes the body less likely to control cancer cell growth. Cancer is the abnormal growth of cells in the body. It is a result of normal cell mutation through its genetic chromosome material, RNA and DNA. Normally cells replicate themselves continually at a rate synchronous with normal growth and repair in a manner specific for its purpose in the body. Cancerous cells multiply faster than normal and lose normal differentiation sometimes forgetting to die.

Chemical and environmental factors may be responsible for 90 percent of all cancers. Elevated risk of cancer from hormone imbalances and toxic buildup in the cells, especially in the colon, can actually be linked to environmental assaults from pesticides and meat hormone residues. While cancer is one of the leading causes of death today, many types of cancer are preventable.

To keep cancer from compromising the body we must strengthen the immune system by naturally enhancing the cellular rejuvenation process. polysaccharides/polypeptides can be a facilitator of this process. As the body's cells become healthier, they will stimulate the immune system and improve its functionality. Also, because polysaccharides/polypeptides balances the pH in the body, the oxygen level is raised. Since cancer *cannot* live in a highly oxygenated environment its survival will be compromised.

Some aggressive forms of cancer treatment often are exceedingly stressful to the body. Side effects can be debilitating, for example, hair loss and the "wasting disease" associated with chemotherapy. Patients using polysaccharides/polypeptides have shown a reduction in the severity of these side effects. Used in conjunction with conventional therapy, polysaccharides/polypeptides can strengthen the immune function and provide a more therapeutic platform for recovery.

"I am forty-nine years old have had rheumatoid arthritis. I have been in the UCLA experimental program on and off for many years, taking a prescription drug to control the pain. I am also afflicted with receding gums, and I visit my dentist every three months to have him check on my condition. One day when I was taking a shower I noticed there was a small lump on my neck. The fear of cancer immediately crossed my mind. The next day I saw my doctor and he told me to have an ultrasound and x-ray on my throat. I was right. It was cancer.

My uncle had been using polysaccharides/polypeptides and suggested it to me. Most of the people know that I am skeptical about new products. But, at this point I had nothing to lose. During my check-up one month later, my doctor was surprised that the lump had completely disappeared and advised that I continue taking the polysaccharides/polypeptides since it seemed to be helping my condition. By the way, my gums are less painful and I am not as tired as I used to be. polysaccharides/polypeptides has helped me at just the right time."

-Linda Arnold, Los Angeles, CA

"I've been taking polysaccharides/polypeptides for a month on the advice of my naturopathic doctor. Prior to taking polysaccharides/polypeptides, I had just quit chemotherapy treatments and my body was greatly debilitated from its side effects. I started a new regimen, which included polysaccharides/polypeptides and noticed that my mood, energy and my feeling of wellbeing has returned. Today I am feeling as good as I felt before contracting cancer. I'm confident that this regime will help me to continue being strong and cancer free."

-Barbara Bankey, Albuquerque, NM

Chapter Eight

Polysaccharides/polypeptides and Chronic Fatigue Syndrome (CFS)

By giving the body the right nutrition, most diseases would be eradicated.
 —Dr. Linus Pauling, Winner of two Nobel Prizes

Most researchers believe that Chronic Fatigue Syndrome (CFS) is a result of mixed infections with several pathogens such as environmental pollutants and chemical contaminants. These contribute to CFS by reducing our immune response, thereby allowing the syndrome to develop. In addition, growing evidence points to the fact that exhausted adrenal glands from high stress lifestyles and an imbalance in the hypothalamic-pituitary-adrenal axis can exacerbate the illness. CFS is a response (or lack of immune response) to the ever-increasing mental, emotional and physical stressors in our environment. As our body's immunity drops lower and lower almost any disruption in our health or emotional state can be the final trigger for Chronic Fatigue Syndrome.[12]

Research indicates polysaccharides/polypeptides can help balance immune system functions in two ways and therefore guard against CFS. A) Polysaccharides/polypeptides can directly and specifically stimulate the immune system by increasing the body's resistance to toxins that may accumulate during the development of infection when the immune system is first called into action. B) Polysaccharides/polypeptides helps to stabilize the hormone cortisol, which is responsible for how we respond to stress. Stress suppresses immunity and destroys our resistance to

---

[12] Fibromyalgia, Lupus, Epstein-Barr virus, and Lyme disease share many symptoms with CFS.

various forms of bacterial or viral attacks. When we are under stress, a great portion of the body's energy is expended. Chronic exposure to stress results in a lowered immune response and decreased health.

"Due to chronic fatigue traced to anemia, in 1999 I retired from being a very active office manager. I consulted with several medical doctors who were unable able to correct the situation. As time passed I became more fatigued and my blood pressure began to rise during exercise or stress. I was under constant medical attention without receiving any appreciable results. I was also diagnosed as being oxygen deprived (to the brain). In July, 2002, I became immobile and had to be placed on oxygen 100 percent of the time. If I removed the oxygen my skin became blue within minutes. In addition, my appetite disappeared, and my stomach began to expand, similar to conditions seen in a starved child in Africa. I was for all practical purposes trapped in my living room by day and by night. I did not see any hope.

In December 2002 I was introduced to polysaccharides and polypeptides. I took the recommended three scoops a day. On the third day I was able to go off the oxygen for a short period of time and make breakfast for my husband for the first time in six months. On the fourth day I was able to go to the shopping mall and have my hair done (two hours without oxygen). On the fifth day I actually cleaned my house. During Christmas of 2002, my family celebrated what I considered to be a miracle.

On the first day of January 2003, only a month after I started taking polysaccharides/polypeptides, I was relying on the oxygen only 5 percent of the time. My appetite was back to normal, my energy returned, and I felt like my old self. I believe that this product will extend my life for many years."
-*Toni Garcia, Albuquerque, NM*

Chapter Nine

Polysaccharides/polypeptides and Hepatitis

The liver is an important organ involved in metabolizing toxins and medications to a less damaging substance. However, in its efforts to protect the body from harm the liver itself may become a victim of toxic exposure and be subject to hepatitis.

Hepatitis is a disease or condition marked by inflammation of the liver. There are several types of viral hepatitis: Type A is a viral infection passed through blood and feces; Type B is a sexually transmitted viral infection carried through blood, semen, saliva, and dirty needles; Type C is a post-transfusion form; and Type D is caused by the Epstein-Barr virus. All forms of hepatitis are characterized by the following conditions: fatigue; flu-like symptoms of exhaustion and diarrhea; enlarged, tender, congested, sluggish liver; loss of appetite to the point of anorexia; nausea; dark urine; gray stools; occasional vomiting; skin pallor and histamine itching; depression; skin jaundice; and cirrhosis of the liver.

Vaccinations are commonly prescribed for Hepatitis, but natural therapies have also had overwhelming success in treating hepatitis cases, both in arresting viral replication, and in regeneration of the liver. Polysaccharides/polypeptides contains properties that can protect the liver from damage and even reverse damage that has already occurred. Polysaccharides/polypeptides works against toxins and assaults that potentially damage the liver and has been found to help protect it from the detrimental effects of hepatitis.

Kiss Your Life Hello with Polysaccharides and Polypeptides.

Chapter Ten

Polysaccharides/polypeptides and Arthritis

> *Let thy food be thy medicine and medicine be thy food.*
> –Hippocrates, the Father of Medicine

Normally considered to be an inevitable part of aging, some schools of thought deem the condition of arthritis to be a result of a toxic body trying to rid itself of waste. When salt combines with other wastes it precipitates out of the blood and lymph fluids, forming abrasive deposits. Ending up in the joints, these deposits may cause a condition known as bursitis and arthritis. Minerals normally carry these deposits out of the body. Our Western diets are deficient in the minerals needed by the body. This is due to over farming of the soil without mineral replacement. Foods grown in this manner (including both supermarket and organic varieties), are lacking the essential minerals needed by the body to function as designed.

Arthritis is one of the long-term effects of mineral imbalance and free radical damage. Mineral imbalance manifests as an acid condition in the body and develops because our pH is not in homeostasis. With specific dietary changes, supplementation with polysaccharides/polypeptides and a good mineral supplement, the pH can be better balanced resulting in arresting the pain and degeneration of even advanced arthritic conditions.

Because polysaccharides/polypeptides is processed from specific rice grains that are grown in highly alkalized and mineralized soil, taking polysaccharides/polypeptides daily will keep the pH of our body balanced. Cleansing and supporting the immune system will also help reduce the effects of arthritis.

"Be patient and polysaccharides/polypeptides will astound you and bring you joy and happiness. I have learned that if it takes five years to get sick, it could take possibly five months to get well. Polysaccharides/polypeptides has made such a great difference in my overall health that I advise everyone to take polysaccharides/polypeptides." With these words Jeff Thompson explains that polysaccharides/polypeptides saved him from a long history of health problems, most significantly, severe arthritis, sinus and hay fever. Relief did not come overnight to Jeff. Indeed, everyone who takes polysaccharides/polypeptides benefits at a different rate—some within hours or days, others within weeks or months. Jeff fell into the latter category.

"My wife, Shamasi and I started taking polysaccharides/ polypeptides in the middle of January 2003. For years she had suffered from arthritis pain in both hands. By the end February her pain was gone. We both are experiencing wonderful results from taking polysaccharides/polypeptides. I've had problems with ulcers and they are gone and what has really surprised me is that my Rosacea (red face) has almost disappeared. I am a true believer in this fantastic product."
-*Jim and Shamsi McMahan, Sugar Land, TX*

Chapter Eleven

Sports Conditioning and Fatigue

Wouldn't it be great if you could perform your favorite sporting activity or exercise program if you wanted? Woefully, those of you who push the intensity threshold of your recreational pursuits often experience a multi-faceted phenomenon known as fatigue. Simply defined, yet physiological quite complex. Fatigue refers to the inability to continue exercise at a given intensity. In all sports and exercise training, the onset of fatigue will vary depending on a person's fitness level, the exercise intensity, and environmental conditions (heat, humidity, and altitude).

The two dominant sport conditioning scenarios leading to fatigue are short-term intense exercise and extended, submaximal training events. Though the physiological mechanisms of these training conditions are distinctly different, their reduction in muscle performance capacity is similar.

Short-term, Intense Sport and Exercise

During vigorous exercise bouts such as sprinting, short burst interval training, and high intensity resistance exercise, continued muscle contraction is dependent on the formation of adenosine triphosphate (ATP) for the demanding energy needs. Under these exercise conditions, there is a glucose breakdown (called glycolysis) that is primarily responsible for maintaining ATP levels. It has been found that during intense muscle contraction; creatine phosphate becomes depleted rapidly, resulting in an incomplete supply of ATP. To make-up for this ATP deficiency, glycolysis increases. However, the increased output of glycolysis results in the accumulation of by-products, including lactate, which has been identified as a potential contributor to fatigue. Lactate production is thought to disturb electrochemical events in muscle cells. Researchers have associated lactate (or lactic acid) production during increased rates of glycolysis with the development of cellular acidosis (decreased pH we commonly refer to as 'the burn') and fatigue.

A neural fatigue also exists during short-term, intensive exercise and sports bouts. Each single motor nerve (meaning under your voluntary control) activates a group of muscle fibers and is collectively referred to as a motor unit. The chemical messengers, or neurotransmitters, that carry the nerve's excitation message to the muscle at the neuromuscular junction, also become impaired with intense exercise. This inhibition results in a decreased efficiency of the muscle fiber's ability to contract.

Extended, Submaximal Sports and Exercise

During prolonged exercises such as cycling, cross-country skiing, and distance running, muscle contraction is also dependent on the ability of metabolic (breakdown of a fuel to release energy) pathways to continuously regenerate ATP. Mitochondrial respiration (aerobic metabolism in the mitochondrion of the cell) becomes the primary supplier of ATP. Decreased levels of blood glucose and low levels of muscle glycogen have been associated with the onset of fatigue in sustained exercise events. Carbohydrates and proteins are necessary for mitochondrial respiration.

Solution

PSP has both polysaccharides (carbohydrates or glucose) and polypeptides (protein or amino acids). By bonding the polysaccharides/polypeptides together under controlled humidity, temperature and pressure, a naturally hydrolyzed alpha-glycan (allowing for 100 percent bioavailability) is formed. Thus, producing an incredibly functional food that when consumed is recognized by the cells of the body as a biological fuel for utilization by the mitochondria to produce the cellular energy or ATP.

*A recent study to show the effect of polysaccharides/ polypeptides on Mitochondrial Function and ATP Production demonstrated a significant increase of ATP in mitochondria metabolism of **54 percent**.

The importance of pH-balancing the body slightly more on the alkaline side than on the acid should be a daily goal. Because PSP is made from a whole food that is grown in an alkalized, mineral-enriched environment, it can facilitate a slightly alkaline pH balance. It efficiently helps to create and maintain a pH-balanced body, which means 'the burn' or lactic acid buildup is greatly reduced.

*PSP also stimulates cognitive enhancement primarily through its influence on important neurotransmitters. These neurotransmitters relay information between neurons and rely on specialized brain chemicals to function properly. Researchers have found that taking PSP will promote rejuvenation and regeneration of the nerve endings.

In-Vitro Mitochondria Cellular Viability/Energy Study (Sawatsri et al.) Royal Thai Army Medical Center, PMK Research Center and, Emory University School of Medicine, Atlanta, Georgia; USA

Energy & Stamina

If having enough energy to earn your daily bread and to get all your chores done is a struggle for you, if you go to bed tired, but wake up even more tired, if you can't get up and go without coffee, or can't slow down and relax without alcohol, or if your fatigue is ruining your mood and your friendships, then it's time to build energy and stamina "The Real Way...the Right Way!"

The Real Way nourishes optimum energy and optimum health by using safe, simple, nourishing whole food complexes (i.e., polysaccharides and polypeptides) and avoiding stimulants.

For powerful stamina and lots of energy, we are well advised to avoid stimulants of all kinds. That means avoiding herb and food stimulants too. It is tempting to try to get more energy by using stimulants. But stimulants decrease overall energy. They provide fast fuel, but no steady flow of energy. Stimulants push us beyond our innate capacity. In effect, they make us work harder than we truly have the energy for, and thus deplete us at deep levels.

The energy-depleting effects of coffee, soft drinks, and white sugar products (including most energy drinks) are cumulative. The more you try to get energy from these sources, the more tired you make yourself. The long-term consequences often include profound fatigue. Black pepper and spices such as cinnamon and cloves are acknowledged stimulants too, and if overused (as in drinking chai daily) can also weaken the internal fires that give you energy.

Herbal stimulants such as ephedra (ma hang), cayenne, ginseng, and guarana are also unlikely to help build real energy and stamina unless used sparingly and wisely. Herbal stimulants may even be quite dangerous, especially when powdered and taken in gelatin caps. Water-based preparations of stimulating herbs (teas and soups) are usually the safest. Small amounts of these herbs taken occasionally are harmless enough. It is long-term use of stimulants that erodes healthy energy.

Authors Note: PSP (a unique combination of polysaccharides & polypeptides) is my favorite energizing natural functional food. It gives me the energy to work all day, write books, train at the gym, and fly all over the world to teach. Because it strengthens the kidneys and the adrenals, it builds powerful energy from the inside out, and gives me, amazing stamina.

Chapter Twelve

Natural Skin Care at the Cellular Level

When it comes to quality skin care products, many people feel if something is natural and nontoxic, it is not strong enough to be effective. Others feel if a product is effective, it cannot possibly be natural. Natural ingredients are not only effective; they are often even more effective than chemicals. The reality is that most skin care manufacturers add chemicals to their products because they are cheaper than the natural, more effective alternatives.

Quality skin care products are built, however, on a strong scientific foundation. Through science we have discovered that skin is not an inanimate object, rather, a complex living organ. Chemicals can harm the skin. Natural ingredients can nourish and heal it.

Several years ago, scientists thought the outer layer of the skin, the epidermis, was made up of flat, dead skin cells that had no interaction with living skin cells. Today, we know this is not true. There are highly active layers within the epidermis featuring intricate interaction between the cells in the epidermis and the growing, lively cells located in the deeper (dermis) layers of the skin. This is hugely significant because if the cells in our epidermis are communicating with cells in the lower layers, we can positively influence the health of our skin on a much deeper level.

The Aging of Our Skin
When does our skin start to age? It is different for each person. Generally, already in our mid 20's the skin's ability to retain water starts to decrease. The oxygen level in the skin also decreases by approximately 25 percent. As a result, skin slowly starts to lose its elasticity, energy, and healthy glow. However, it is never too early to start using intensive anti-aging skin care.

More serious signs of aging appear in our 30's. The skin starts to produce less collagen, which causes formation of mimic wrinkles. Those are deeper than just dry lines and are harder to get rid of. The creation of new cells in the skin slows down. This results in a dull, tired complexion. Other skin aging factors include smoking, stress, free radicals, bad diet, not enough exercise or sleep etc.

In our 40's, the skin becomes drier, thinner, and as a result, more fragile and susceptible to the formation of wrinkles and damage by free radicals. Spots will appear, as will discoloration or freckles, making the complexion uneven.

Over 50, the decreased production of estrogen and progesterone will cause the skin to become still dryer, thinner and more sensitive. It is believed that decreasing estrogen levels can cause increased collagen to break down, resulting in more wrinkles, loss of firmness and sagging. That sounds like some awfully bad news. But there is some good news, exceptionally good news. There is a lot that can be done about our skin and the aging process.

The Good News: Bioavailable Polysaccharide and Polypeptides
PSP (Polysaccharide/Polypeptide) administered topically is 100 percent bioavailable. Bioavailability means that there is total absorption at the cellular level. It has been shown to penetrate to the deep layers of the skin and regrow collagen, elastin, and proteins, thereby restoring a more youthful appearance to the skin, reducing wrinkles, and eliminating age spots. PSP also stimulates skin cell communication, protects against free radicals, and speeds up cell regeneration. It veritably turns back the clock, making our skin healthy, radiant, youthful, and supple.

"I am a Master Esthetician and was introduced to PSP just over a year ago. It is by far my favorite skin care product. The results are incredible. I don't know of another skin care product that you actually apply to your skin and consume. I believe it's so effective because it works from the outside in and the inside out! I love that PSP is so simple to use and so effective. It's truly AMAZING!"
-*Ashley D. Las Vegas, NV*

"For many months I have had the problem of reactions in the skin of my face, because of different external things: shaving, sun, pollution, cold weather, etc. It stated with a" small rush " in the form of white or red patches . The doctor told me it was normal for precisely the reasons that I expressed. I began to apply myself PSP on my face while I shared the opportunity to the owner a beauty salon, she offered me a treatment to eliminate these abnormalities in the skin of my face. I agreed, but demanded that only use PSP on my treatment For six days I underwent treatment wet cleaning, application of PSP and after 20 minutes I withdrew it with water. Results were immediate, the skin regains its normal color, white spots and red spots disappeared, but more importantly, recovered smoothness and softness. I'm sure PSP, restored the skin of my face."
-*Luis Alfonso Lozano Lecompte, Bogotá Colombia*

Kiss Your Life Hello with Polysaccharides and Polypeptides.

Chapter Thirteen

Research and Studies[13]

Polysaccharides/polypeptides (PSP) may prevent neuron vulnerability in human neuroblastoma cells (preliminary, unpublished data).
-*A study by Dean, M. Ishak, PhD,MD, College of Complementary Medicine, Malaysia*

Abstract (Preliminary data)

Objective: The current study investigated the neurotrophic and neuroprotective action of a unique formulation of Polysaccharide/polypeptides, which consists of carbohydrate, crude protein, and essential minerals by using pressure and mechanical hydrolysis to make a complex formulation.

Methods: Using neuronal cell lines prepared from the LA-N-5 (Los Angeles Neuroblastoma) for Alzheimer's disease (AD) in complete media and treated with indicated manner, inverted microscopic evaluated morphological and biochemical analysis were conducted to determine the neurotrophic and neuroprotective properties of polysaccharides/polypeptides .

Results: Results of this analysis demonstrated that polysaccharides/polypeptides significantly decreased neuronal cell death, a cellular marker of memory formation. Dose response analysis (experiment going on) indicated that the lowest effective concentration of polysaccharides/polypeptides exerted the minimal neurotrophic effect. Results of neuroprotection studies demonstrated that polysaccharides/polypeptides induced highly significant

---

[13] The formulation used in the testing was polysaccharides/polypeptides

neuroprotection against beta-amyloid, peroxides, and glutamate induced toxicity.
Discussion: Abnormality of glucose/energy metabolism shows relation to AD (1,2,2,4). Polysaccharides/polypeptides may prevent impairment of glucose/energy metabolism and may improve the ability of neurons to reduce the levels of free radicals (scavengers) and thereby affect ATP levels. (11,12).
Conclusion: polysaccharides/polypeptides S induced cellular markers of memory function in neurons critical to memory and vulnerable to negative effects of aging, cellular degeneration and Alzheimer's disease. Results of the current study could demonstrate the cellular mechanism of polysaccharides/polypeptides on cognitive function and a possible intervention in Alzheimer's disease.
Key Words: Polysaccharides/polypeptides, Cell Death, Alzheimer's disease (AD), Neuroprotective.

Introduction
1.1 Alzheimer's disease: A scientific mystery and major impact. Abnormality of glucose/energy metabolism shows relation to Alzheimer's disease (1,2,3,4). Degenerative and cell death are major causes in AD.
1.2 Polysaccharides/polypeptides is a complex formulation that consists of carbohydrate, crude protein and essential minerals by using pressure and mechanical hydrolysis to make a complex formulation designated polysaccharides/polypeptides (5).
1.3 Polysaccharides/polypeptides is very safe because it contains phytochemicals that have components of carbohydrates, crude protein and essential minerals by using pressure and mechanical hydrolysis to make a complex formulation designated polysaccharides/polypeptides. Evidence by observation from animal (pig) data showed that polysaccharides/polypeptides could decrease morbidity from Ataxia (polysaccharides and poly-

peptides may improve cerebral blood flow). In clinical use we found that polysaccharides/polypeptides improves short and long-term memory (6).

1.4 LA-N-5 (Neuroblastoma cell lines) have been used for model of Alzheimer's disease *in vitro* (7,8,9,10).

Control: Nerve cells

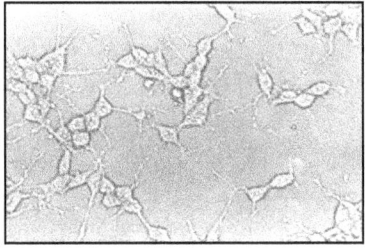

Same nerve cells injured by beta-amyloid neurotoxin.

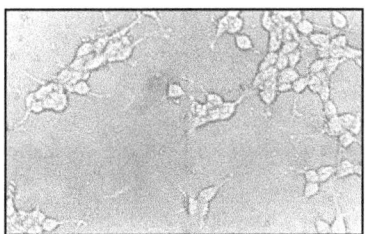

Same nerve cells rejuvenated
after being pretreated with polysaccharides/polypeptides

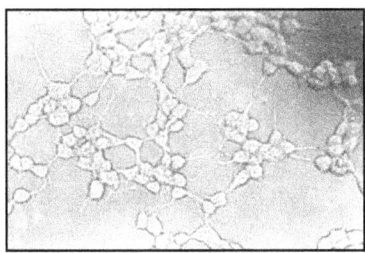

Objectives
1. To determine if polysaccharides/polypeptides (PSP) may promote neurotropic and neuroprotective actions that show decreased cell death (Apoptosis) in the Alzheimer model *in vitro*.
2. To determine if polysaccharides/polypeptides shows neurotrophic and neuroprotective action in AD model and to determine what is the mechanism of polysaccharides/polypeptides.

For proposed mechanism of polysaccharides/polypeptides induced neuroprotection in AD model *in vitro*.

Materials and Methods (1)
1. Neuronal culture
   Neuronal cells lines were prepared from the LA-N-5; Los Angeles Neuroblastoma derived from bone marrow metastasis of four-month-old male patient. Cells were propagated in RPMI 1640 supplemented with 10 percent FCS, 2mM glutamine, 50 IU/ml penicillin, 50 ug/ml streptomycin, and 1 ug/ml fungizone (complete medium).
2. Morphological analysis
   By using inverted microscopic evaluated morphological analysis of LA-N-5 in indicated conditions.
3. Neuronal
   Neuronal viability was determined by inclusion criteria of trypan blue.
4. The neurotrophic and neuroprotective action of PSP
   was determined by inducing other neurotoxic substrates as indicated conditions.
       1.1 Estrogen deprivation exposure: Neuronal viability was determined by estrogen deprivation exposure.
       1.2 Hydrogen peroxide exposure: 1uM H_2O_2 for 5 minutes at 37 deg. C. During exposure, E2 or

PSP was added concurrently with H2O2. After 5 min. the culture was rinsed two times with HBS, and Fresh medium with E2 or PSP was replaced.
1.3 Glutamate exposure: 0.2 uM Glutamate 20 min. at room temperature.
1.4 Beta amyloid25-35 exposure: 8 ug/ml AB25-35 24. at 37 deg. C.

Results
* Neuroprotection by polysaccharides/polypeptides against other neurotoxic results:
- Estrogen deprivation induced neurotoxicity
- Hydrogen peroxide induced neurotoxicity
- Glutamate induced neurotoxicity
- Beta amyloid25-35 induced neurotoxicity

* Dose dependent of PSP shows neuroprotection against other neurotoxins

Discussion
Abnormality of glucose/energy metabolism shows relation to AD (1,2,3,4). polysaccharides/polypeptides may prevent impairment of glucose/energy metabolism and may improve the ability of neurons to reduce the levels of ("scavenger") free radicals and thereby affecting ATP levels (11,12).

Conclusions
- PSP contains a unique formulation consisting of a complex form of carbohydrate, crude protein and essential minerals by using high pressure and mechanical hydrolysis to make a complex formulation designated polysaccharidepeptides which in vitro, has con-

sistently demonstrated that it prevents cell death from other neurotoxicity agents.
- PSP induced cellular markers of memory function in neurons critical to memory and vulnerable to negative effects of aging, cellular degeneration and Alzheimer's disease. Results of the current study could demonstrate the cellular mechanism of PSP on cognitive function and a possible intervention in Alzheimer's disease.
- In clinical application, polysaccharides/polypeptides may promote cellular mechanism in memory and neuronal survival and may be used as a nutritional supplement in aging, cellular degenerative processes and a possible use for preventing Alzheimer's disease.

References
1. Blass, JP, Gibson, GE, Shimada, M, Kihara, T, Watanabe, M, and Kurinioto, K, (1980) "Brain carbohydrate metabolism and dementia," *Biochemistry of Dementia* (Burman, D. and Pennock, C.A., eds.), Wiley, London, pp 121-134.
2. Blass, JP, Sheu, KFR, and Cederbaum, JM, (1988), "Energy metabolism in disorders of the nervous system," *Rev. Neurol. (Paris),* 144, 543-563.
3. Beal, MF, (1992), "Does impairment of energy metabolism Result in excitotoxic neuronal death in neurodegenerative Diseases?" *Ann. Neurol.,* 31, 119-123.
4. Blass, JP, Sheu, KFR, and Tanzi, R, (1996), "a-Ketoglutarate dehydrogenase in Alzheimer's disease in Energy Metabolism," *Neurodgenerative Diseases (Fiskum, G, ed.),* Plenum, NY, pp. 185-192.
5. Laboratory report from Pacific Lab Services, Report No: /396-3971/LS/2001, Feb. 19th, 2001.
6. Interview with Medical Doctors Testimonial No.007, 018, 058 and 068.
7. Preuss, U, Mandelhow, EM, (1998) "Mitotic phosphorylation of tau protein in neuronal cell lines resembles phosphorylation in Alzheimer's disease." *Eur J Cell Biol,* 76 (3): 176-84.
8. Mesco, ER, Timiras, PS., "Tau-ubiquitin protein conjugates a human cell line," *Mech Ageing Dev* 199; 61 (1): 1-9.
9. Davis, PK, Johnson, GV, (1994) "Monoclonal antibody Alz-50 reacts with bovine and human ser albumin," *J Neurosci Res,*; 39(5): 589-94.

10. Fabrizi, C, Businaro, R, Lauro, GM, Starace, G, Fumagalli, L, (1999) "Activated alpha2 macroglobulin increase beta-amyloid (25-35) induced toxicity in LA-N-5 human neuroblastoma cells," *Exp Neuro,l,* 155(2): 252-9.
11. Beal, MF, (1995), "Aging, energy, and oxidative stress in neurodegenerative diseases," *Ann. Neurol,* 38, 357-366.
12. Mattson, MP, (1994), "Mechanism of neuronal degeneration and preventive approaches: Quickening the pace of AD research," *Neurobiol. Ageing* 15, (Suppl.2) S121-S125.

Report on Possible Solutions in the Global Health Problems (April 2002)
-Dr. Mohamed Ahmed, M.D., President of Association of Complementary Medicine, Malaysia

The present food consumed by people in developed countries is predominantly processed food treated with pesticides, insecticides and soil nutrients of chemical nature. The introduction of many different chemicals into the body along with the food we consume has interfered with normal functioning of cells both at their intrinsic and extrinsic functions. It is now known that many proteins fold up into abnormal forms, called Rogue Proteins. These abnormal forms can be the cause of a multitude of diseases.

Example: The underlying reason why Alzheimer's and Creutzfeldt-Jakob diseases cause dementia is because small clusters of Beta Amyloid molecules—the misfolded protein—disrupt the junctions between nerve cells in rat brains. (Prof. Denis Selkoe of Harvard Medical School and colleagues.)

While scientists are trying to produce Synthetic Peptides (called Synthetic Mini-Cheperonin) to destabilize the abnormal folding of the protein, new research appears to dismiss attempts to treat the diseases by attacking the deposits and instead indicates that scientists must try to prevent the proteins misfolding in the first place.

Researchers believe that they have found the secret to correct this misfolding of proteins and sugar at the cellular level. Research in-vitro tests on neuronal cells shows that polysaccharides/polypeptides is able to protect the neurons from toxic materials like Beta Amyloid, Peroxides and Glutamate.

Hypothesis is that polysaccharides/polypeptides is able to provide the polysaccharide and polypeptide necessary for normal protein and sugar folding, thus enabling cellular repair.

Clinical studies in the form of *evidence-based studies* prove the hypothesis. Numerous testimonials and "clinical study results" have encouraged the scientists and clinicians to indulge further into research.

With the support from the Ministry of Science and Technology of Thailand for the research projects, scientists will move even faster. More research, both in-vitro and in-vivo, is ongoing to further prove and to publish more findings. This natural food, in its simplest form, has the solution for most of the modern ailments. Instead of wasting millions of dollars on high tech surgery and medicines, we should turn to natural food, for solutions to the global problems.

Diabetic Study with Polysaccharides/polypeptides Bangkok, Thailand Oct. 2003
-Dr. Mohamed Ishak M.D, Dr. B. Chalermporn M.D., Dr. Mark D. Smith N.D.

Introduction: Type 2, adult-onset, non-insulin dependent diabetes, affects about 85 percent of diabetics, striking one in 18. With its complications, it is the third leading causes of death in the U.S. It's a chronic degenerative disease in which disturbances in normal insulin mechanisms impair the body's ability to use carbohydrates. Type 2 diabetics produce insulin, the hormone that helps convert food into energy, but isn't used properly (insulin resistance), causing glucose to build up in the bloodstream, depriving cells of the nutrients they need.

Test subjects: 702 individuals that were diagnosed with Type 2 Diabetes, by a physician. The volunteers were given polysaccharides/polypeptides to take three times a day for 90 days. They were tested at: 0 days, 30 days, 60 days, and 90 days.

Final Results: 570 out of 702 people completed all four laboratory tests: before taking polysaccharides/polypeptides 30 days, 60 days, and 90 days after taking polysaccharides/polypeptides. 84.22 percent had improvement within 30 days 89.65 percent had improvement within 60 days 90.18 percent had improvement within 90 days.

Preliminary Efficacy Study of polysaccharides/polypeptides in Multiple Sclerosis (Feb. 14 2003)[14]

-Mark Dargan Smith, N.D., PhD., Dean, University of Natural Medicine, New Mexico

Introduction

Multiple sclerosis (MS) affects 350,000 Americans. With the exception of trauma, it is the most frequent cause of neurological disability beginning in the early to middle adulthood age groups. MS is twice as common in females as in males and its occurrence is unusual before adolescence. A person has an increased risk of developing the disease from the teen years to age forty with the risk gradually declining thereafter.

MS is considered an autoimmune disease, whereby the body's own immune system (which normally targets and destroys substances foreign to the body) mistakenly attacks normal tissues. In MS, the immune system targets the brain and spinal cord, the two components of the central nervous system.

The most common symptoms of MS include:
- fatigue (most common), mental fatigue, drowsiness

---

[14] The formulation used in the testing was polysaccharides/polypeptides

- tingling, numbness, tremors
- sudden onset of paralysis
- loss of balance, coordination, dizziness & lightheadedness
- weakness in one or more limbs
- blurred or double vision; optic neuritis
- slurred speech; swallowing problems
- slowed thinking, decreased concentration & memory

Methodology & Test Subjects
Three volunteers were chosen. Each was diagnosed by a physician, suffered from Multiple Sclerosis for a multitude of years and was in a very degenerative condition. The volunteers were given polysaccharides/polypeptides to take three times daily for a period of 30-60 days.

Patients #1 & #2 had blood urine Oxidative Stress Profiles completed at days 0, 30, & 60. They filled out symptom questionnaires at days 0 & 30. It was not necessary to complete a 60-day post-test symptom questionnaire as they had few symptoms remaining at that point.

Patient #3 had a day 0 & 60 blood and urine Oxidative Stress Profile completed and also filled out the symptom questionnaires at days 0 & 60. All results are included in this clinical report. The following are the protocols that were adhered to.

Protocol
1. Test subjects met the following criteria:
    - No age limitation
    - Experiencing all of the following:
      Medical diagnosis of Multiple Sclerosis.
      The conditions or imbalances on the MS questionnaires (Each patient had been diagnosed with chronic degenerative Multiple Sclerosis).
1.2 Duration of study: 0, 30, & 60 days pre- and post-testing

1.3 Pre- and post-testing was performed as follows:
- Interview for qualification
- Physical and symptom evaluation
- Completed a pre and post physical and symptom assessment form
- Completed a MS questionnaire, before and after
- Pre and post Oxidative Stress Panel (blood and urine).

1.4 Intake (Diet, medication and supplementation).
- Maintained: current eating habits, medications, vitamins, other supplements
- Variable compliance on food elimination: dairy products, sugar, caffeine, alcohol and tobacco for duration of the study (optional)

1.5 Lifestyle
- Maintained current lifestyle
- Avoided long distance air travel

1.6 Patients completed Informed Consent Form
1.7 Dosage: 5 grams (1 tsp.), 3 times a day
1.8 The physical, symptom and laboratory measures were all completed
1.9 Inclusion/Exclusion criteria was followed

Laboratory Results

In one patient, who also had diabetes (type 2), self-testing indicated that there was a significant decrease in blood sugar from over 200, down to the low 100's on a consistent basis. This could be due in part to current research demonstrating that the addition of SOD (superoxide dismutase) and catalase to cultures of pancreatic islets exposed simultaneously to alloxan resulted in a partial restoration of insulin synthesis.

Polysaccharides/polypeptides delays the production of Single Molecule Sugar (Glucose). This delay will slow down the increase of the sugar in the blood, while the amino acids will help the pancreas secrete adequate insulin, so sugars are brought to the cells at a more efficient rate, thereby, bringing normalcy in the blood sugar level.

The patients did not perform any internal body cleansing or detoxification procedures to enhance the elimination of toxins, which would have been the recommended protocol.

Conclusion
All three individuals participating in the study experienced significant reductions in their Multiple Sclerosis related symptoms. A reduction in degenerative disease-causing free radicals and an increase in antioxidants such as SOD (superoxide dismutase) and the glutathiones were demonstrated in the Oxidative Stress Profiles. As the SOD antioxidant increases were almost triple in the first thirty days and then declined afterward, it would most likely be attributed to the metabolism of the free radicals, a metabolic balancing, or any of the reasons previously suggested in this study.

One of the patients (with diabetes) experienced immediate and continued improvements in blood sugar regulation.

Patients experienced a normalization of weight (decrease in obesity in one and maintaining of weight in others who did not wish to lose weight).

The results of this study along with the in-vitro research would demonstrate cellular protection from particular neurotoxins known to have a deleterious and degenerative effect on all nerve cells, (i.e., beta-amyloids, glutamates, and peroxides). The nutrients in the polysaccharides/polypeptides would also provide the cellular fuel necessary for cellular communication and regeneration.

References
1. Laboratory report from Pacific Lab Services, Report No: /396-3971/LS 2001 Date: February 19th, 2001.

2. Mesco, ER, Timiras, PS, "Tau-ubiquitin protein conjugates in a human cell line," *Mech Ageig Dev*, 1919; 61(1): 1-9.
3. Beal, MF, (1995), "Aging, energy, and oxidative stress in neurodegenerative disease," *Ann.Neuro, 38, 357-366.*
4. Mattson, MP, (1994), "Mechanism of neuronal degeneration and preventive approaches," *Neurobiol Aging,* 15(suppl.2), S121-S125.

Glitch in Power-Generating Mitochondria Could Upset Amyloid Processing and Cellular Regeneration (March 2003)
-Dr. Bruce Yanker, M.D., Associate Professor of Neurology, Harvard Medical School

In the general population, Alzheimer's disease strikes an individual at a relatively late age, even though Mild Cognitive impairment, a potential precursor to Alzheimer's, is now found to occur at all ages. In those people with Down's syndrome the disease is more unforgiving. Most people with the syndrome develop Alzheimer's pathology by late middle age, including deposits of the plaque-forming protein amyloid-beta that are often more severe than in most other Alzheimer's patients. Why the two diseases are intimately linked is unclear. Research suggests that a malfunction in the mitochondria of Down's syndrome patients may be to blame. The resulting loss in cellular energy may explain how amyloid-beta slowly clogs the brain and why Alzheimer's is a disease of aging.

Impaired mitochondria may be to blame for the early onset of Alzheimer's disease in people with Down syndrome. This may be a result of an extra copy of chromosome 21, which can lead to the over expression of certain proteins. The amyloid precursor protein, which has been cleaved to form amyloid-beta, and presumably its increased production contributes to the early onset of Alzheimer's.

Specific cells with diminished mitochondrial function can accumulate the pathogenic form of amyloid-beta. A switch from the protective form to amyloid-beta could be dangerous to the cell. In culture, Down's syndrome neurons die off relatively quickly, but the team research found that a recombinant form of the protective amyloid precursor fragment could effectively rescue this degeneration.

Amyloid-beta itself comes in two sizes—the longer form is thought to be more pathogenic and toxic, and more likely to form plaque. Down's syndrome cells are in this pathogenic form, which is the direct precursor of the senile plaques. Researchers found that the trafficking of the amyloid-beta protein was also significantly altered in certain Down's syndrome cells. Normally it is quickly shuttled out of the cell once it is produced. But, in Down's syndrome cells the amyloid-beta remained inside the cell, localized in the organelles of the secretory pathway through which the precursor protein is normally trafficked. Furthermore, the protein accumulates in highly insoluble lumps.

The processing, trafficking, and folding of proteins is powered by ATP, which is generated in the mitochondria. Accumulation of amyloid-beta is due to abnormal protein folding of the amyloid-beta protein once it's generated in the cells, due to loss of energy metabolism. Current findings provide a link between mitochondrial dysfunction that normally occurs in the aging brain and the predisposition to Alzheimer's. Mitochondrial dysfunction may trigger the accumulation of amyloid-beta, which impairs neurons and eventually kills them

Research has shown that feeding mitochondrial metabolites to aged rats can help slow the signs of age-related decay, suggesting a therapeutic angle on targeting the mitochondria in diseases of aging.

Authors note: Polysaccharides/polypeptides stimulates the mitochondria with the necessary metabolic fuel to not only thwart the development of the toxic amyloid-betas, but also to aid in the regeneration of new cells. This process may prevent brain cell degeneration and symptoms associated with Alzheimer's and other Neurological diseases.

Neuroprotective Effect of Polysaccharides/polypeptides in Cell Lines Models of Alzheimer's Disease (march, 2006)

-*Dr. Nel Sidell, Emory University School of Medicine, Atlanta, GA*

Alzheimer's disease (AD) is associated with extensive loss of specific neuronal subpopulations in the brain. This disease is characterized by the presence of numerous extracellular plaques and tangles, a primary component of which is a 39-43 amino acid peptide know as beta-amyloid. Although progress has been made in defining cells that are vulnerable in this disorder, the cellular and molecular changes preceding neuronal loss and the underlying etiology remain undefined.

A number of studies have suggested that certain vitamins/nutrients, through their antioxidant properties, can counteract reactive oxygen species (ROS)-dependent cytotoxic effects on neural cells, thereby protecting the cells against insults that give rise to AD pathology. The purpose of the study is to test the ability of one such nutrient, polysaccharides/polypeptides, to prevent oxidative and beta-amyloid induced cytotoxicity of human neuroblastoma (nb) cell lines as in-vitro models of AD.

Statistical analysis:
Data were analyzed using Student's test measuring the cells viability of experimental groups compared with control groups.

Discussion:
The percentage of cells viability of neuroblastoma cell at 1.33 mb/ml of a polysaccharides/polypeptide increased 54 percent. "The Student" test found that the percentage of cells viability at 0.33 mg/ml with polysaccharides/polypeptide (experimental group) and a control group were significantly different.

Conclusion:
The polysaccharides/polypeptide shows dependent for neuroprotective effect in AD model and has an optimal effect by increasing ATP in mitochondria metabolism 54 percent. It definitely has a role to intervention in AD and other conditions.

Nature, Time and Patience (three great physicians)

Nature has managed to produce what man can only try to copy—polysaccharides/polypeptides, is a truly beneficial combination of balanced nutrients. As a functional food it has an effect on our body's systems without harmful side effects.

In most cases, experiencing healthful benefits by taking a functional food, polysaccharides/polypeptides, takes time. Our body needs our patience. As we are gentle to our body by breathing correctly, eating good nourishing foods, taking a functional food, polysaccharides/polypeptides, drinking clean water and exercising moderately, we will soon notice our body saying "Thank You" in return.

So, how soon can someone expect to see and fee results? This varies from person to person, and it depends a lot on what condition we are hoping to improve and how much we are taking each day. In general, it depends on ho undernourished we are at the cellular level. The more our immune system is compromised, the longer it will take. Remember that we arrived at the point of cellular communication deficiency after years of questionable eating and suboptimal lifestyles. We need to be patient to see the results we hope for.

Chapter Fourteen

Frequently Asked Questions

Several questions in this section pertain to the supplement polysaccharides/polypeptides where results have been qualified verifying its efficacy.

Q. How are the polysaccharide/polypeptides different from other available polysaccharidepeptides (i.e., those found in mushrooms)?

A. The polysaccharides/polypeptides are the only known Alpha-Glycans, which means the structure is so small that they can be assimilated 100 percent by the body and therefore be totally absorbed into the cells. Other polysaccharide/peptides are beta-glucans, which are larger molecules and cannot be totally assimilated into the cell. Alphaglycanology assures that polysaccharides/polypeptides possesses the functional characteristics that are needed to be recognized by the DNA and RNA.

Q. How do polysaccharides/polypeptides work?

A. polysaccharides/polypeptides positively influence the body by inducing an anabolic (building) phase and creating a reduction in the catabolic (breakdown) phase in order for the body to correct the metabolic disorders which are largely responsible for most degenerative health problems. Some of the underlying symptoms of metabolic disorders include:

- free-radical attack
- Hyper-Insulinemia
- toxic colon
- hypoanabolic phase
- Metabolic Oxidative Stress
- abnormal genes
- impaired detoxification
- hypercatabolic phase

- Leaky Gut Syndrome
- Hyperlipidemia

polysaccharides/polypeptides formulations are designed to enhance the body's natural healing processes by stimulating the mitochondria to produce ATP, allowing DNA repair to take place.

Q. What can the functional food polysaccharides/polypeptides do which other products cannot?
A. The best source for cellular function is a high, bioactive form of essential elements that improve the cellular environment to create a harmonious basis for ultimate gene expression. It has been proven that polysaccharides/polypeptides can work both in-vitro and in-vivo to correct degenerative health problems at the cellular level.

In-vitro studies show its efficacy in preventing injuries of neuronal cells from neurotoxins such as beta-amyloid, glutamate, and peroxides. In-vivo studies show that within ninety days, at a dosage of one measured scoop per day taken in the morning, polysaccharides/polypeptides is able to reverse the blood chemistry profile of individuals suffering from many kinds of cardiovascular and degenerative disorders. These include high cholesterol, high blood sugar, high triglycerides, high SGOT/SGPT, low in RBC, WBC and platelets counts.

Q. Is polysaccharides/polypeptides safe for pregnant or lactating women?
A. Because polysaccharides/polypeptides is a form of a whole food complex, it may provide all the basic nutrients needed by most women. Although polysaccharides/polypeptides has not caused any problems in pregnant or nursing women, they are asked to consult with their physician before taking polysaccharides/polypeptides as they would for any supplement.

Q. Can polysaccharides/polypeptides be taken along with medications and will it interfere with the efficacy of medicines if they are taken together?
A. Reports of adverse reactions have not been forthcoming from physicians who administer polysaccharides/polypeptides together with medications. Doctors, who have had experience using polysaccharides/polypeptides along with their medication programs, including chemotherapy and radiation, have observed faster recovery from illnesses in their patients. Patients that have been on polysaccharides/polypeptides for a period of time may ask their doctor to readjust their medication, often lessening the dosage and/or eliminating the medication entirely.

Q. Who would benefit the most from taking this all-natural food?
A. Studies show daily intake of this natural whole food product can be extremely beneficial to the brain function. People who are suffering from degenerative diseases such as Alzheimer's, Multiple Sclerosis, and Parkinson's benefit the most. People suffering from arthritis, diabetes, high blood pressure, high cholesterol, strokes, attention deficit disorder and hyperactivity, and Tourette's syndrome greatly benefit from polysaccharides/polypeptides.

Q. Will I go through a "healing crisis"?
A. A healing crisis is when the body's natural defense systems are waging war on the illness itself and is trying to purge the illness from the body. People whose systems are quite toxic may go through a healing crisis. During this time, symptoms may worsen. However, this healing crisis will normally only last a few short days and when over, the body heals very rapidly. Improvements in health will be extremely noticeable. The healing crisis can be uncomfortable but once it has passed people have been astounded at how well they begin to feel. In all cases polysaccha-

rides/polypeptides has produced positive results that have been observed in a time period ranging from a few days to as many as twelve weeks, normally averaging four to eight weeks.

Q. Can healthy people take polysaccharides/polypeptides ?
A. polysaccharides/polypeptides is particularly valuable to individuals whose bodies are subjected to more than the usual "wear and tear." That includes those who exercise regularly, and those who are exposed to environmental stress in today's world. Modern lifestyles forces most people to live under stress, leaving them little or no time manage their health. Supplementing with polysaccharides/polypeptides is important for our modern society even if they believe they are healthy.

Q. Are polysaccharides/polypeptides safe for pets?
A. Because polysaccharides/polypeptides is not species specific it can be given to your pets without any problem. Sprinkle a little into their food, depending on the size of the animal and encourage them to drink plenty of water. Pets will benefit in exactly the same way as humans.

Chapter Fifteen

Professional Citations[15]

If any man can convince me and bring home to me that I do not think or act aright, gladly will I change; for I search after truth, by which man never was harmed. But he is harmed who abideth on still in his deception and ignorance.
　　　　　　　　　　　　　-Marcus Aurelius Antoninus

"From my own clinical observation, polysaccharides/polypeptides can be safely recommended for chronically ill individuals who suffer from neurological disorders ranging from Alzheimer's, Parkinson's, Multiple Sclerosis, Meningitis, Myasthenia Gravis diseases and also stroke patients. Faster recovery was observed when polysaccharides/polypeptides was given along with other forms of treatment and medications. Significant improvements in the symptoms of these patients have clearly been seen."
-*Mohamed Ishak Syed Ahmad, MD, PhD, President Association of Complementary Medicine, Malaysia*

"I have been using the supplement polysaccharides/polypeptides on twenty-four patients that had multiple medical problems including gastro-esophageal reflux, irritable bowel syndrome, gastritis, and diabetes. I have been quite satisfied with the response. My patients find polysaccharides/polypeptides soothing, safe and it appeared to quiet their gut inflammation. I feel this product enhances GI healing and improves digestion from the anecdotal responses I have received."
-*Norton L. Fishman, MD, Center for New Medicine, Rockville, MD*

---

[15] The supplement PSP was used by the professionals cited in this chapter. Therefore, their comments are specific to that product.

"I have been in family practice for many years. During that time, I have seen many conditions benefit from a nutritional program. My first interest in nutrition began after seeing a Chronic Fatigue patient get tremendous relief from using various herbs, although I didn't know much about herbs at the time. However, due to the great results we received I started to study the wonderful means of enhancing health through nutrition. The more I read, the more I realized that even though medicine is a viable way of helping the sick, proper nutrition is a must.

Many products claim they are all natural, yet, on the label it mentions binders, fillers, and preservatives, which are far from natural. I searched for something truly all natural and after reading information on polysaccharides/polypeptides I realized this was the answer for my patient's various problems. I have always wanted a good nutritional product that I could recommend to my patients and their families. polysaccharides/polypeptides is the perfect solution. polysaccharides/polypeptides is a great product for the whole family. We even give polysaccharides/polypeptides to our pets."
-*George Michaels, DC, Los Angeles, CA*

"I'm a registered nurse and have been diagnosed with chronic high blood pressure, atrial fibrillation and post-traumatic, post-operative osteoarthritis in my right knee. While I'm generally receptive to new ideas, I am usually cautious when someone introduces me to a new 'cure-all' product.

I started taking polysaccharides/polypeptides on January 12, 2003. Prior to that date, I was on three blood pressure drugs (blood thinners) and potassium replacement for my cardiovascular problems. I was also taking medication for my knee pain. I was so focused on the potential cardiovascular benefits of polysaccharides/polypeptides, that I didn't realize that my knee had been pain-free all week, despite the frigid cold and rainy weather.

Needless to say, I stopped taking *Celebrex* and my knee remains virtually pain free.

In the meantime, I ran out of my blood pressure medications. I do not recommend that anyone stop taking any of their medications without consulting their physician and I do take my blood pressure daily. But, what I saw happening was indeed a miracle! In the past, if I needed blood pressure medication for more than two doses, I would see a dramatic increase in my pressure. Since taking polysaccharides/polypeptides, in spite of not being on one of my medications, my blood pressure stays in the normal range. No combination of my prescribed medications has ever maintained a normal pressure before. I can't wait to see my cardiologist's face on my next visit. Polysaccharides/polypeptides may not be the cure, but I love my new polysaccharides/polypeptides tune-up!"
-*Marsha Slocum, RN, Sugar Land, TX*

"Polysaccharides/polypeptides is the new generation of natural super foods instantly recognized by the DNA. polysaccharides/polypeptides creates cellular energy that remedies an unbelievable number of degenerative conditions, such as: Alzheimer's, MS, cancer, AIDS, Parkinson's, Hyperactivity, Heart Disease, Diabetes, and most metabolic disorders. It is good for all ages and can improve memory function, cellular repair, blood sugar, skin conditions, hormonal function, fatigue and libido."
-*J. Toan, MD, Director, Cho-ray Hospital, Vietnam*

"My father, who at 81 years-old, was diagnosed with fourth-stage Hepatic Cancer in mid-February 2003. He had been bed and wheelchair ridden prior to and when taken to the hospital. When he was admitted he was experiencing severe pain throughout his body, especially in his bones. Upon admission, the doctors placed him on fluid therapy (electrolyte imbalance). Other symptoms he exhibited included high fever, pre-coma condition, edema and lack of energy,

The PET scan showed enlarged liver to 11x6 cm (standard size 11x11 cm). His cancer cells had migrated to the Lymphatic system. My father was told that he had only three more months to live and was released to go home because there was no further treatment available. No medication was prescribed except antipyretic drugs. But due to black color stool-bleeding the medication was stopped.

After my father was released from the hospital, I had him start taking polysaccharides/polypeptides . Three weeks later the following happened: edema subsided; most of the pain disappeared; he can now walk and do normal routines; regained appetite for food; and he has much more energy. He went back to the hospital for another check-up and the doctor discovered his liver enzymes greatly improved. As a medical doctor I am a firm believer that many people can benefit by taking polysaccharides/polypeptides ."

-*S. Sek, MD, Bangkok, Thailand*

"As a practicing physician in the field of holistic medicine I have observed significant improvements in many patients with cognitive impairment and Parkinson's when taking polysaccharides/polypeptides. In fact, I would not have any reservations in recommending this product both as a preventive measure and an alternative treatment for anyone suffering from neurodegenerative disease."

-*Dr. Kampon Sriwattanakui, MD, Bangkok, Thailand*

"I have not experienced another product quite as effective as polysaccharides/polypeptides in remedying such a variety of illnesses and conditions. Its benefits for the entire gastro-intestinal system have been astounding. I have seen direct results in its usage for diabetes, MS, intestinal dysbiosis, gastric ulcers and from

constipation to diarrhea. polysaccharides/polypeptides seems to decrease the radical damage and increase the anti-oxidants in the body."
-*Mark Dargan Smith, ND, PhD, Dean of the University of Natural Medicine, Santa Fe, NM*

"In my practice I use polysaccharides/polypeptides to manage a variety of conditions, Tourette's, Parkinson's, Alzheimer's, and ADD/ADHD. I advocate using whole foods instead of multiple supplements. The body can heal itself and a whole food product, such as polysaccharides/polypeptides, supports the healing process. I have noticed in myself an increase in metabolism. I have lost several inches around my waist. The biggest improvement has been my eyesight. I do not have to use my glasses for distance and for reading. Cardiovascular disease and high cholesterol are quite common in my family. Even though my diet is healthy, and I take the various supplements that I wrote about, my cholesterol had been around 250-265. Since I began taking the product my cholesterol decreased to 215, my ratio (HDL: LDL) is 3.3 and my ratio was 5.4. All my other numbers were in the normal range. I am now in the category of a lower risk of heart attacks. Polysaccharides/polypeptides is and will continue to be in my daily regimen."
-*Author: Howard Peiper, ND, Albuquerque, NM*

"I am a Master Esthetician and was introduced to PSP just over a year ago. It is by far my favorite skin care product. The results are incredible. I don't know of another skin care product that you actually apply to your skin and consume. I believe it's so effective because it works from the outside in and the inside out! I love that PSP is so simple to use and so effective. It's truly AMAZING!"
-*Ashley D. Las Vegas, NV*

Kiss Your Life Hello with Polysaccharides and Polypeptides.

Chapter Sixteen

User Testimonials*

> *He that hath a truth and keeps it,*
> *Keeps what not to him belongs.*
> *But performs a selfish action,*
> *And a fellow mortal wrongs.*
> —Andrew Jackson Davis

*The supplement polysaccharides/polypeptides was used by the people who are cited in this chapter. Their results are specific to that product.

Conditions treated within this chapter:

Attention Deficit Disorder	Hip problems
Autism	Hyperactivity
Back Pain	Hypertension
Blood Pressure	Leg Pain
Cancer	Lupus
Carpal Tunnel	Migraines
Cerebral Palsy	Osteoporosis
Chronic Fatigue	Overweight conditions
Colitis	Parkinson's
Diabetes	Rosacea
Down's Syndrome	Seizures
Eczema	Skin
Fibromyalgia	Sports
Gangrene	Stroke
Goiter	Tourette's

Alzheimer's

"I am a firm believer of polysaccharides/polypeptides and wouldn't be without it myself as a preventives and for total energy. My 89-year young father who suffers from Alzheimer's and a stroke he endured a year ago, has benefited from polysaccharides/polypeptides more than anyone. He is now walking and talking, writing letters that we can read and has gained thirty-four pounds (he was skin and bones after his stroke). My mother, 87-years young, also has benefited from taking polysaccharides/polypeptides. She was diagnosed with Fibromyalgia and was suffering mostly 'foggy' days. Now, I can never find her, she is traveling and visiting and seldom has a 'foggy' day. Thank you! Thank you!"
-Lori Ware, San Diego, CA.

Autism

"I have a three-year-old autistic child who has been seen by numerous doctors that specialize in autism. Their suggestions availed nothing. Then a friend of mine told me about polysaccharides/polypeptides and the remarkable results it was having on autistic children. Since our child has been taking polysaccharides/polypeptides, (we also take it), the doctors are totally amazed. There is literally no sign of her having autism. She is a normal child, interacting and playing with other children. I hope and pray that other parents who have autistic children read this and start taking polysaccharides/polypeptides."
-Nancy Perlito, CA

Back Pain

"A severe whiplash from a car accident eight years ago gave me chronic neck and lower back pain. Consequently, I have suffered from lower-space-disc disease and have found that just lifting five to ten pounds is very difficult. After taking polysaccharides/polypeptides three times a day for only one week, I could

pick up my two and one-half year-old grandson, who weighs thirty pounds, without any pain. I am so excited; I am telling everyone!"
-*Hilarie Crone, York, PA*

Blood Pressure
"Four years ago, I was diagnosed with high blood pressure. My doctor had me on four medications. Even with these medications my blood pressure sometimes reached 180/100. I have lived in fear of a heart attack during recent years. I was introduced to polysaccharides/polypeptides during the first week in December 2002. I began a protocol of taking one scoop three times a day. On January 1, 2003, I checked my blood pressure and was shocked to find that it was 126/64. This is considered a low reading for me. My doctor has now reduced the dosage of all my medications. One day I know I will be able to eliminate them. Praise the Lord for P polysaccharides/polypeptides. I now have a future to look forward to."
-*John Doak, El Paso, TX*

High blood pressure
"High blood pressure runs in my family "My blood pressure in September 2002 was 144/90. I have only been taking polysaccharides/polypeptides since January 2003 at two doses a day, and my blood pressure has dropped to 128/73. This improvement is very encouraging to me.

Meanwhile, my husband had open-heart surgery in January 2003. Postoperative blood work revealed that he had high cholesterol, high blood pressure and high triglycerides. The doctor advised him to get his counts down immediately or he would be right back in the hospital with more blockage problems. I started him on polysaccharides/polypeptides as an adjunct to his regular medications and gave our physician information on the product. After one and a half months of him being on polysaccharides/polypeptides three times a day, I was anxious to have his

blood work redone. The results subsequently revealed that all his counts were either significantly lowered or within normal limits: Cholesterol went from 244 to 127; Triglycerides from 471 to 221; and the Chol/HDL ratio from 6.10 to 5.08. His blood pressure is also down to normal. Well, needless to say our family doctor was quite surprised and even shocked with the results after such a short time. He asked us for additional information on polysaccharides/polypeptides. Under his doctor's supervision, I am now working towards weaning my husband totally off his medications."
-*Betty Atland, York, PA*

Colon Cancer
"In August 2001 I was diagnosed with colon cancer. I had an operation and was put on chemotherapy treatments. Later on, I was diagnosed with Parkinson's disease and suffered from tremors, dizziness and chronic fatigue. In May 2002 I started taking polysaccharides/polypeptides and over the course of about one year I observed fewer problems with my tremors. The symptoms of dizziness and chronic fatigue have disappeared. My immune system is back to a healthy state, even after having chemotherapy."
-*Phrakru Tien (Thai Monk), Bangkok, Thailand*

Carpal Tunnel
"My name is Morrie Louden. I've been a professional Bassist (Musician) for thirty years. I got carpal tunnel syndrome about four years ago from having to play my standup bass six days a week. It was serious enough to have surgery. The surgery improved the situation a bit, but the pain was still there. I began using polysaccharides/polypeptides. After the first week, the pain had subsided. Five weeks later I realized I was now capable of working steady and have gone back to playing six days a week without a bit of pain. WOW! I wish I'd have known sooner about

polysaccharides/polypeptides. It would have prevented having my surgery!"
-*Morrie Louden, Austin, TX*

Cerebral Palsy

"My son, who has Cerebral Palsy, has been taking polysaccharides/polypeptides for three months. The most immediate change that we noticed in my son was his improved digestive system. He had been very constipated. We have also noticed that he is much more alert and are pleased with the results in this short time."
-*Pam Oliversen, Seattle, WA.*

Cerebral Palsy

"Fatin was born in 1995 and was diagnosed with Cerebral Palsy. Since birth, she has suffered from stunted growth, physical weakness and was always sick. With so many neurological deficiencies she was difficult to manage. We tried everything from medicines to herbs and various forms of supplements, but we saw no improvement in her condition. In October 2000 when Fatin was five and one-half years old, we started to give her polysaccharides/polypeptides and noticed rapid improvement with her neurological functions. She started to sit and stand (with some assistance), something she was not able to do before. She became more alert, started to understand what was being said to her, and was more responsive. Nowadays, she seldom gets colds, flu, or fever. As of February, 2002 Fatin has grown stronger and her interactions with others have been miraculous. We will continue to give her polysaccharides/polypeptides ."
-*Shamsuddin Malik, Fatin's father, Johore, Malaysia*

Chronic Fatigue

"I have been suffering from Chronic Fatigue Syndrome for many years. My naturopathic doctor suggested that I start taking a unique whole food formula from Thailand. He had learned that

this amazing whole food was helping others who had various immune-suppression ailments. Since taking polysaccharides/polypeptides my energy level is better, my aches and pains are gone and my immune system is stronger."
-*Marge Smith, Albuquerque, NM*

Diabetes
"I was diagnosed with Type II Diabetes in 1998. I am a very large lady and have had poor results with many diabetic prescriptions. My blood sugar was 160 when, on January 15, 2003 I started taking polysaccharides/polypeptides . After two days my blood sugar dropped to 140—a miracle! On January 17th, only four days after starting polysaccharides/polypeptides, my blood sugar was 118! This is nothing short of awesome!"
-*Beverly Peasley, Elizabethtown, KY*

Dialysis patient
"I have been a dialysis patient for three years and am currently undergoing the procedure three times per week. Ever since I started the dialysis, my skin turned dark, I lost my energy, and I felt constantly fatigued. I had to rest for an hour after being on the dialysis machine. My feet were swollen and numb from retaining fluids causing me many sleepless nights.

After taking polysaccharides/polypeptides for only two months, I noticed the following changes: my skin went back to its original color; I could do housework without feeling fatigued; and I was able to get up and walk immediately after each dialysis. I now sleep well through the night, and I am certain that by taking v, my dialysis frequency will someday be reduced."
-*Lee Sen, Melaka, Malaysia*

Down's Syndrome
"When my son, Abraham was born, it was an amazingly easy delivery, and his features were remarkably normal. It wasn't until

after his first three-month inoculations that he started displaying symptoms of Down's Syndrome. For Abraham's first two years, I did the best that I could to provide a nutritional program. I kept him off wheat, dairy and sugar products. But Abraham's appetite was poor, and he wasn't walking or talking. He had a short attention span. A friend of mine introduced me to a product called polysaccharides/polypeptides that had anecdotal studies helping with Down's Syndrome. I started to give him polysaccharides/polypeptides and the first thing that I noticed was his appetite improved. Within a few weeks, Abraham began standing and taking steps. His muscles grew stronger, and his focus and attention span was also improving. After only ten months on polysaccharides/polypeptides Abraham is not only walking, but he is running like a normal child. During his last motor skills testing, he has advanced to a two-year-old level. He holds focus on an activity up to thirty minutes (rare for a Down's Syndrome child). I can't tell you how thrilled we are with Abraham's progress."
-*Mariam Stein, Escondido, CA.*

Eczema

"Since her birth, my daughter, Mei Jin, had never had a restful day or even a restful night due to itchy lesions. After she had been on polysaccharides/polypeptides for nine weeks, I noticed that 80-90 percent of her eczema lesions slowly had disappeared. I thank the people who introduced to me polysaccharides and polypeptides. I no longer use antibiotics or steroids on Mei Jin's skin."
-*Lim Mei Jin, Mei Jin's mother, Singapore*

Eczema

"A friend of mine introduced me to PSP for my husband who had severe eczema.. I started giving him one pack a day and, in a short time his skin cleared up and remained that way for many weeks. However ,the eczema reappeared but thankfully not nearly as severe as before and only on his arms and a little on his legs.

I consulted with Dr. Howard Peiper and he explained that my husband is detoxifying one layer at a time. Now, several months later, his eczema is totally gone…..Thank You PSP!"
-*Helen Miller, Marquette, MI*

Fibromyalgia and colds
"I use polysaccharides/polypeptides for my fibromyalgia and irritable-bowel syndrome. I was so pleased with how I felt that I decided to give my son a half scoop of polysaccharides/polypeptides every day. He had been suffering constantly from a runny and a stuffy nose. Now he no longer suffers. If he does get a cold, he only gets a runny nose if I forget to give him polysaccharides/polypeptides a few days in a row."
-*Sherry Adams, AZ*

Gangrene
"I have suffered with Diabetes for eleven years. I now also have neuropathy, retinopathy and nephropathy. Because of a sore on my right ankle, I developed an ulcer that turned into gangrene. My wound was not responding to medication and the doctors suggested amputation (below my knee). I started taking polysaccharides/polypeptides three times a day along with ozone treatment. I also applied polysaccharides/polypeptides locally to my wound. My diet has been controlled through eating high protein foods and eliminating carbohydrates. I eventually got off my insulin. Within a short period of time, all edema around the wound settled down and I was able to walk short distances. My doctor had me finish taking a course of antibiotics and stated that my wound was healing extremely well. When I returned for the next appointment, a skin grafting was scheduled. Thanks to polysaccharides/polypeptides, I can now play basketball and jog. What a gift!"

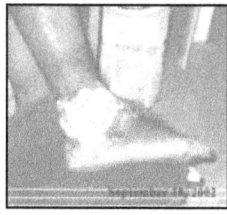 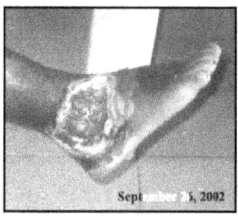 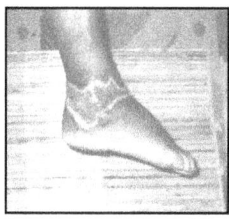

September 18. 2001   September 26, 2002   October 29, 2002

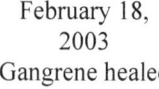 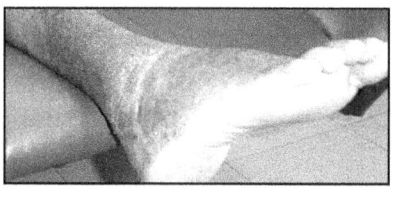

February 18, 2003
Gangrene healed

-Mohamed Zain, Prof. of Engineering, University Tech of Malaysia

Goiter

"I have suffered from abnormal thyroid function for the past seventeen years and have had a goiter on my neck for this entire period. Doctors advised me to have an operation and for some reason I refused. polysaccharides/polypeptides was introduced to me and within three months my goiter greatly reduced its size. Now it is just about gone. I am glad my intuition told me that there was an alternative to surgery."
-Tak Koh, Singapore

Hip Replacement

"I started taking the polysaccharides/polypeptides product in February, 2003, in preparation for a total hip replacement that was to take place in April. I had the surgery and was discharged three days later a day earlier than expected (usually patients that have had total hip replacements must stay for four or five days after surgery). Two weeks after discharge from the hospital I started taking the polysaccharides/polypeptides product every day. In only a few weeks, I could easily go up and down stairs and walk over a mile just for fun. My physical therapist report read 'doing extremely well.'

The therapist told me that my recovery would most likely be 40 percent faster than the typical hip replacement patient—which means 40 percent less expensive to me. I'm 59-years old and have invested my professional life in being a health care economist and medical practice consultant. Taking polysaccharides/ polypeptides has been the best health care investment I've ever made. I believe the polysaccharides/polypeptides product could have significant benefits towards lowering health care costs."
-*Clifford Todd, Newport Beach, CA*

Hip Dysplasia in a dog.
"I ordered P polysaccharides/polypeptides for my husband who is diabetic and who is getting remarkable results. So, I thought about giving polysaccharides/polypeptides to my eight-year-old German Shepard, Heidi who has hip dysplasia. In about one week I noticed she was moving better. She was going up the stairs without help or making sure someone was behind her when she did. She also has more energy. I just put about a quarter of a scoop of polysaccharides/polypeptides in her food once a day."
-*Candella Shaffer, Dallas, TX*

Hyperactivity
"My seven-year-old son Jesus has had hyperactivity problems since he was three years old. Jesus was very easily distracted, unable to count to more than forty and to maintain concentration on any subject. Most of the time, I couldn't put him to sleep. He used to watch TV until one o'clock in the morning. After about a month of taking polysaccharides/polypeptides, we noticed Jesus was able to count to four hundred or more without losing concentration. He can count by fives up to two hundred sixty. His teach-

er told us that he is now one of the most behaved students in the class. He now goes to sleep at 8:00 P.M."
-*Anna Dominguez, Soledad, CA*

Hypertension, hyperthyroidism

"I've suffered from hypertension, hyperthyroidism and have been overweight for about thirteen years. Because of poor night vision, my driving has always been bad while driving at night. Since taking polysaccharides/polypeptides, my vision has improved, and I've also lost fifteen pounds. My doctor told me that my blood pressure and my thyroid are now normal. I don't take hypertension and hyperthyroid medication anymore. These improvements were observed only after a few months on polysaccharides/polypeptides, taking it three times a day."
-*Dodi Cruz, Bellwood, IL*

Leg Pain and Diabetes

"I have experienced severe pain in my left leg since I had back surgery in 1991. My doctors told me I had irreversible nerve damage. This was unwelcome news to anyone, but especially for a person who had insulin-dependent diabetes. The pain made it difficult to walk. Two weeks after I started taking polysaccharides/polypeptides , the pain subsided enough that I stopped taking pain pills. My doctor was amazed. Since taking polysaccharides/polypeptides, I have been able to reduce my insulin from 32 units a day to 18 units."
-*George Stein, NY*

Liver illness

"My baby was born premature at eight months with a severe illness in the liver. She also was not moving nor crying, so the doctors placed her in an incubator for ten days. The hospital eventually allowed me to take her home. The prognosis was not good. A friend of mine suggested giving her polysaccharides/polypeptides. Within two days, my husband and I noticed she started moving

her head, crying, and making noises. We took her to see the doctor for a checkup and he was amazed. He told us to continue feeding her polysaccharides/polypeptides. She is now one year old, healthy, strong, and happy as any normal child.
-*Nelly Romero, Monterrey, Mexico*

Lupus
"My son, who is 13-years old, has been diagnosed with LUPUS for the past ten years. I was introduced to a whole food complex, polysaccharides/polypeptides. I started to give my son one teaspoon per day. Recently, I took my son to the Lupus specialist and the eye doctor (my son was also losing his sight because of Lupus). Both doctors told me that his vision was again normal and the recent test results showed the Lupus condition was totally gone."
-*Antonio Garcia, Monterrey, CA.*

Multiple Sclerosis
"I have had Multiple Sclerosis and elevated blood sugar problems for many years. I am wheelchair bound. In 1986 I experienced weakness in my hands, and I was hospitalized with a blood sugar crisis. I was in the VA hospital for a month. I have quadriplegia, greater in my legs and on my left side. I have lost more than two-thirds of my muscle strength. My SOD (antioxidant) level was 1,542, which was below standard.

Only thirty days after I started taking a food supplement called polysaccharides/polypeptides, my SOD level went up to 3,158 and I can tell you that now my feet are much healthier. They are not as red or swollen as they used to be and are looking normal. I had stiffness, mostly in my left ankle and knee— now I am more mobile. My thighs also are not as stiff, and I notice I am developing more muscle on them. The strength in my arms and legs has improved. I used to let my care provider push me all the time in my wheelchair when we were out, but now I push myself most of the time.

I went to the barbershop a few days ago and for the first time I could get off the electric scooter and into the barber chair by myself. Before, two men had to help me up. I have also lost quite a few pounds during this short time. I am grateful to polysaccharides/polypeptides for turning my life around."
-*Francisco Gabaldon, Santa Fe, NM*

Multiple Sclerosis

"For many years, I suffered with "MS brain fog" and had to work hard to think well. I could not decide if it was from MS (Multiple Sclerosis) or the beginning of a senile dementia. The severe headaches continued off and on and MS fatigue continued. I had too little energy to even consider walking around a large grocery store. It was customary for me to be in bed eleven to twelve hours a night and not awaken refreshed. My SOD (antioxidant) level was 1,728.

Thirty days after I started to take polysaccharides/polypeptides daily, I felt considerably better. My SOD level had doubled to 3,766. Each day I recognized significant improvement. I no longer wear an ankle brace for support, something that I had done for years. I have not had any spasticity in my legs and back since taking polysaccharides/polypeptides. Also, the edema in my legs is markedly less and they look nearly normal. Other changes I had observed included greater bladder control as well as a reduction in my medication (Synthroid) that was prescribed for a hypothyroid condition.

I now can do physical things that I could not do during past years. The oppressive multiple sclerosis fatigue is nearly gone. My support group said at this month's meeting that I looked years younger, and I was walking very well. I am thrilled at the return of near normal health and look expectantly each day for new improvements."
-*Janice South, Santa Fe, NM*

Osteoporosis

"While having my annual physical exam three years ago at the age of forty-three, I decided to be tested for bone density. The results determined I was a high risk for osteoporosis. I was surprised because I am regularly active, take nutritional supplements and consider myself in excellent health. Then I started taking polysaccharides/polypeptides, faithfully. I began noticing a lot of improvement in my mental focus, memory recall, my skin and hair and my stamina while exercising. This past July, I went for another bone density test. The nurse from my doctor's office called me surprised. The results were normal. I really believe taking polysaccharides/polypeptides has helped me and will continue helping me prevent osteoporosis".

-*Gina Scott, Laguna Nigel, CA.*

Overweight and allergic

"I used to weigh 250 pounds and have suffered from a stuffy nose and skin allergies for many years. I could not work long hours due to fatigue and tiredness. After one month of taking polysaccharides/polypeptides , my vitality has come back. I don't tire as easily as I used to. I can now work longer hours and even my bowel movements have greatly improved."

-*Maria Dominguez, Soledad, CA*

Parkinson's

"I have had a serious problem with Parkinson's disease. The last six months I have not been sleeping very well. Even after taking sleeping pills, I could not sleep very long, sleeping just two to three hours at a time. I was introduced to polysaccharides/polypeptides in March of 2002. The first week I only took the polysaccharides/polypeptides one time a day. Then I started taking polysaccharides/polypeptides three times a day and began getting great results. I now sleep without any sleeping pills for six to eight hours. I feel rested and energetic when I

wake up in the morning. My friends that know me are amazed at how well I look."
-*Jose Zuniga, Tijuana, Mexico*

Pseudo Bowel Obstruction

"My daughter has a rare medical condition called pseudo bowel obstruction in which the muscles and nerves in her small intestine do not function properly. She is on antibiotics regularly for bacteria overgrowth in her GI tract. Before taking polysaccharides/polypeptides, she was not doing well and totally dependent on IV nutrition. When she tried to eat by mouth she would get very ill. The first week on this functional food, she began eating almost full calorie by mouth some days. We were eventually able to give her a 26-day break from her antibiotics and motility medication. Another amazing thing we've noticed, a few months after taking this product is that her multiple surgery scars have lightened up in color to where it almost matches the rest of her skin. She also has had an improvement in some nerve hearing loss that was supposed to be permanent. My daughter continues to struggle with her rare illness. However, I know the polysaccharides/polypeptides have had a positive difference and give her many good days."
-*Laura Brock, Kingsford, MI*

Rosacea

"I went to see my mother who is forty-nine years old and suffers from Rosacea, which is also known as adult acne. Rosacea affects 14 million Americans today and can be treated but not cured. It causes facial swelling and redness with visible signs of blood vessels. She has been fighting Rosacea for several years. I gave her the polysaccharides/polypeptides and within one week the Rosacea was barely noticeable. She is only taking one scoop a day. We can't wait to see what the next thirty days will bring."
-*Casey Minshew, Houston, TX*

Skin

"For many months I have had the problem of reactions in the skin of my face, because of different external things: shaving, sun, pollution, cold weather, etc. It stated with a" small rush " in the form of white or red patches. The doctor told me it was normal for precisely the reasons that I expressed. I began to apply myself PSP on my face while I shared the opportunity to the owner a beauty salon, she offered me a treatment to eliminate these abnormalities in the skin of my face. I agreed but demanded that they only use PSP in my treatment. For six days, I underwent treatment: wet cleaning, application of PSP and after twenty minutes I withdrew it with water. Results were immediate, the skin regains its normal color, white spots and red spots disappeared, but more importantly, recovered smoothness and softness. I'm sure PSP, restored the skin of my face."

-*Luis Alfonso Lozano Lecompte, Bogotá Colombia*

Sports

I've found that PSP is the product *every* athlete dreams of finding. It has not only given me an amazing increase in both energy and endurance but has brought me to a higher level of overall performance. PSP has improved my physical and mental health to the point that I've had 20-year-olds asking me how I've managed to make such dramatic changes! I now find that my immune system is so much stronger that I no longer catch the colds that many surfers endure. My doctor was so impressed with my physical condition that he's now reduced much of my regular medication. Now, I'm finding yet another fantastic use for PSP... my skin! You can imagine the damage the sun has done to my skin from 30+ years of constant exposure. I now apply it to both my face and hands every day. My skin is now much smoother and softer, plus it just *glows*!"

-*Ellen Petrus, California*

"I found my career as a dance instructor worked extremely well into my family life until I began to have severe pain in my knees. I was unable to jump, run or do aerobic exercise without pain. As a dance instructor, these are skills you must not only possess, but do them explosively. One of my students recommended taking PSP. I was astonished to find that the pain in my knees disappeared after only a month. That, plus the extra energy and sense of wellbeing."
-*Julie, Mexico*

"I regularly compete in High Performance Cycling at the MASTER level (for 40-50-year-olds) and generally average biking over 75 miles per day. Before learning about PSP, I had tried, without success, countless natural products to achieve better performance. I can definitely say that since taking PSP my performance has more than doubled! The additional energy and stamina has been so tremendous that I am now able to compete in younger categories with 20-30-year-olds."
-*José Garza López*

Stroke

"On January 11, 2003 I was introduced to polysaccharides/ polypeptides, and it has changed my life! Five years ago, a blood clot traveled to my brain and caused a stroke. After eighteen months of speech, physical and occupational therapy, I was showing little progress and I no longer qualified for services. All therapy was stopped.

The left side of my body was affected from the stroke as was my speech and ability to walk. I have had little use of my left arm, and my left hand had remained in a fist position. I have always been a lefty and by not having the use of the left hand I have had to deal with a big adjustment. I was always tired and needed to sleep a lot. I never felt energized.

I started taking polysaccharides/polypeptides on the evening of January 11 in the amount of three times a day. Several wonderful things happened. My left arm was no longer contracted— it was hanging down by my side in a relaxed, natural position (this is the arm that has not been straight in years). I could voluntarily open and close my left hand and I could even hold a deodorant bottle in my left hand! My speech and my thinking both were notably clearer. I now sleep very well at night and actually look forward to getting up, in fact, I am up to thirty sit-ups every morning! I still take an afternoon nap, but I do not require the sleep I did before I started taking polysaccharides/polypeptides .

Other people are noticing the difference in me. They cannot always pinpoint what is different; they just say I looked great! I had only been on this product sixteen days and I knew firsthand what it could do. I am my own testimonial. Thank you for polysaccharides/polypeptides. The last two weeks have been so remarkable. I am truly looking forward to the months ahead. Who knows what the total outcome will be?"
-*Jim Nicholson, Maynard, IA*

Stroke

"My wife, Neyda, is sixty-eight years old, and suffered a severe stroke in July 2001. She was in a coma for more than eighteen days. The doctors predicted that she would be bed- and wheelchair-bound for the rest of her life. The left side of her body was paralyzed. She could not express herself nor recognize her family. She had to be helped with all her needs including eating.

In the spring of 2002, she started taking polysaccharides/ polypeptides three times a day. After only six weeks, she was able to stand and take steps. She had movement and control over her left side of her body. She had started to exercise and take physical therapy. She also began to lift a weight of one pound with her left leg and arm, both of which had been previously paralyzed.

I had witnessed her progress with my own eyes every time I visited her. Her doctors and relatives were amazed with her progress. The prognosis is favorable that she may recover almost completely from her stroke."
-*Jose Matos, San Juan, PR*

Tourette's syndrome
"Haley, my nine-year old daughter, was diagnosed this summer with Tourette's, a condition that causes uncontrolled muscle movements. Haley's tics were mainly facial. She'd also gasp for air when she was excited or upset. Drugs are prescribed for Tourette's but because of their terrible side effects we decided against them.

ADHD (attention deficit hyperactivity disorder) is associated with Tourette's, and Haley was also experiencing trouble concentrating in school and at home. When she was frustrated with herself, the tics would worsen.

I was introduced to polysaccharides/polypeptides and hoped this was the answer to my prayers. I started her on one dose a day in the morning and within four days her dad and I both noticed her tics were gone! We just couldn't believe it happened so quickly. Therefore, we assumed it was just a fluke. Then after a week and still no tics, we started believing it was the polysaccharides/polypeptides. We asked Haley if she felt different and she said yes. She explained she was having an easier time concentrating at school and other kids didn't distract her as easily as before. We are noticing she minds better at home and doesn't forget things at school as she previously had done.

Her tics came back during one period in her recovery, and we discovered the reason; she wasn't taking all of her polysaccharides/polypeptides in the morning! Now we are closely monitoring her to make sure she gets the full dosage. When she follows the recommended dosage her tics go away. I can't thank the people enough

who introduced polysaccharides/polypeptides to me. It has truly changed Haley's life and ours as well."
-*Linda Lutz, Haley's mom, Minneapolis, MN*

Author's note: *I have written two best sellers on ADD/ADHD and have found that over 50 percent of the children that are on Ritalin for hyperactivity actually have Tourette's. Ritalin aggravates Tourette's syndrome.*

Visual and hearing problem – Down's Syndrome
"Our 40-year-old Down's Syndrome daughter was enrolled in an enabled arts program for three months. We had to withdraw her from the program as her personality changed for the worse and her speech regressed so bad we could hardly understand her. She has a hearing visual problem. After several weeks we decided to try polysaccharides/polypeptides (which I have been taking for my Type II Diabetes with a tremendous amount of success). Within three days we started noticing a change. She started vocalizing more clearly and talking about people in her past eighteen years ago. She seemed so much happier we couldn't believe it. She recently had her eyes examined and her prescription was reduced significantly, and her hearing problems have 'disappeared.' We are so grateful to have our daughter back, thank you so much."
-*Evelyn Malmen, Albuquerque, N.M.*

Conclusion

> *Let no one presume to give advice to others that has not first given good advice to himself.*
> –Seneca

    The information and statistics from the previous chapters will mean nothing to you unless you take action. This is more than a book about polysaccharides/polypeptides . It is a book about people like you—individuals who are in search of health and natural healing. The people who told their personal stories all felt that polysaccharides/polypeptides had changed their lives. For some, it was miraculous, and for others it was significant enough to make the quality of their lives much better. polysaccharides/polypeptides is a product unlike any other. You deserve the best quality of life, health, and wellness and polysaccharides/polypeptides can restore and preserve that health for a lifetime.

Kiss Your Life Hello with Polysaccharides and Polypeptides.

Resources

Polysaccharides/polypepeptides are available in a variety of forms. However, all forms are not *alpha-glycan* processed. Below is my recommendation:

The Original Cellular PSP™
Marketed by PSP marketing Inc.
(866)-777-5050
Or contact your local distributor:

Bibliography

-Anderson, Nina, Peiper, Howard *Secrets of Staying Young*, Safe Goods Publishing, 1999.

-Bell, Rachel, Peiper, Howard, *The ADD & ADHD Diet,* Safe Goods Publishing, 2001.
-Ishak, Dr. Mohammed, "Possible Solutions to the Global Health Problems*," Nature's Journal,* April 2002.
-Khalsa, Dharma, *Brain Longevity*, Warner Books, 1999.
-Page, Linda, *Healthy Healing, 11th Edition,* Traditional Wisdom, 2000.
-Natures Journal #444, p. 632-636, 2001.
-Humphries, Courtney, "Glitch in Power-generating Mitochondria could upset Amyloid Processing and Cellular Regeneration," *Harvard Research*, Feb 2003.
-"Healing Hepatitis Naturally," *Dr. Rx for Healthy Living*, Freedom Press, 2000.
-Ishak, Dr. Mohamed M.D, Chalermporn, Dr. B. M.D., Smith, Dr. Mark D., N.D.
-Peiper, Howard, *Naturopathic Secrets of Your pH,* Natures Publishing, 2002.
-Wise, SJ, *The Sugar Addict's Diet,* Safe Goods Publishing, 2000.

Other Books by Safe Goods

Natural Eye Care Series: Macular Degeneration
Natural Eye Care Series: Glaucoma

Natural Eye Care Series: Cataracts

Natural Eye Care Series: Dry Eye

Natural Brain Support

The Shattered Oak

A Barnstormer Aviator

Flying Above the Glass Ceiling

Spirit & Creator (Spirit of St. Louis)

Letters from My Son

Nutritional Leverage for Great Golf

Overcoming Senior Moments Expanded

Prevent Cancer, Strokes, Heart Attacks

Cancer Disarmed Expanded

Eye Care Naturally

Velvet Antler

Efficacy of Velvet Antler In Veterinary Practice
www.SafeGoodsPublishing.com

Author

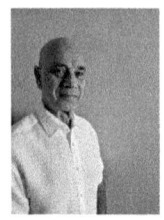 **Dr. Howard Peiper, N.D.**

Howard Peiper N.D, is a Doctor of naturopathic medicine. While beginning his career in optometry, he was immediately drawn to the field of alternative health. In 1972, he received his degree in Naturopathy. After a decade in private practice, Dr. Peiper moved on to become a successful consultant, speaker, and writer. Over the years, his cutting edge articles have appeared in numerous medical journals and magazines. He also serves on the medical advisory board for several nutritional companies. Dr. Peiper has written several best-selling titles including *The ADD and ADHD Diet* and *New Hope for Serious Disease*. He is a frequent guest speaker on radio and television and has hosted his own radio shows including the award-winning TV show, Partners in Healing. Currently, Dr. Peiper lives in the Tampa Bay area and continues to travel and lecture throughout the world.

www.ingramcontent.com/pod-product-compliance
Lightning Source LLC
LaVergne TN
LVHW011727060526
838200LV00051B/3053